————————THE INTERNATIONAL MANUAL OF————————
HOMOEOPATHY & NATURAL MEDICINE

An introduction to the basic principles of homoeopathy and
ayurvedic medicine, with easy to follow remedies for a variety of
ailments, and general guidelines for healthy living.

THE INTERNATIONAL MANUAL OF
HOMOEOPATHY
&
NATURAL MEDICINE

Principles of an age-old
practice of alternative medicine,
with step-by-step remedies.

Dr C.H. Sharma
(Edited by David Leland)

THORSONS PUBLISHING GROUP
Wellingborough · New York

Published in the UK by Thorsons Publishers Ltd.,
Denington Estate, Wellingborough, Northamptonshire NN8 2RQ
and in the USA by Thorsons Publishers Inc.,
377 Park Avenue South, New York, NY 10016

Thorsons Publishers Inc. are distributed to the trade by
Inner Traditions International Ltd., New York

First published in 1975
Second edition (revised, reset and enlarged) 1985

British Library Cataloguing in Publication Data

Sharma, Chandra H.
   The international manual of homoeopathy
   and natural medicine. — 2nd ed.
   1. Pharmacy, Homoeopathic
   I. Title   II. Leland, David
   III. Sharma, C. H. Manual of homoeopathy
   natural medicine.
   615.5'32   RX671

ISBN 0-7225-1142-6

Printed and bound in Great Britain

ABOUT THE AUTHOR

Dr Chandra Sharma was born in Vaso in the Gujarat district of India. His childhood was a mixture of two cultures as he was brought up in both India and Africa, during which time he learned how to speak Gujarati, English and Swahili.

At the age of 14 he went to Japan to study dentistry after which he decided to study medicine in India. In 1941 he qualified as a doctor in Bombay and, after extensive general practice in Indian hospitals, he came to Europe to specialize in the study and treatment of the diseases of women and children. Soon after arrival he became seriously ill with what was diagnosed as an incurable disease of the spinal column. However, he was completely cured by homoeopathy after which he found that he could no longer practise orthodox medicine with conviction. He therefore studied and qualified as a homoeopathic physician.

Having found homoeopathy to be wanting in certain aspects, he extended his studies into psychology under Jung at the Jung Institute in Switzerland. He also studied and researched other unorthodox therapies such as osteopathy, Chinese medicine, nature cure and radiesthesia.

In 1950 he won a Nuffield scholarship to America where he added further qualifications at various post-graduate institutes and was also made a Fellow of the Emerson University Research Council.

After serving in American hospitals he returned to Europe, and in 1953 became a member of the Centre Homoeopathique de France. In 1974 he founded with J. G. Bennett the Ramana Health Centre which is devoted to alternative medical treatment and research into alternative medical techniques. He is at present Medical Director of 101 Private Clinic and is also Dean of the Register and Council of Homoeopathy. Dr Sharma has written several books and lectures extensively all over the world.

David Leland's first introduction to homoeopathy was as a patient and he has since become a lay-student of the subject. He has worked extensively in films, television, theatre and as a writer and also a director and actor.

CONTENTS

FOREWORD BY J.G. BENNETT

This is no ordinary book and the opportunity to contribute a foreword is a privilege I gladly accept. Dr Sharma is far more than a successful homoeopathic physician. He has penetrated deeply into the medical systems of East and West. This combined with his own original research work and his vast clinical experience has given him a rare insight into the bases of health and disease that he seeks in this book to share with others. He has not written a treatise on homoeopathy for the practising physician, but rather an introduction to the fundamentals of natural healing addressed as much to the interested layman as to the specialist. It is also a work book that everyone can use.

We are so accustomed to think of 'science' as the creation and prerogative of the West, that we are astonished to discover how many of the greatest discoveries were made by the Arabs, the Chinese and the Indians. European scientists like Dr Joseph Needham have taught us that there are still unsuspected treasures to be found in Eastern science and medicine. In some respects, Eastern medicine is still far ahead of ours and we should be foolish to disregard it. Dr Sharma set himself to master the principles and techniques of both Eastern and Western Schools of Medicine and has shown that armed with this great wealth of experience, a physician can do far more to keep his patients healthy than would be possible with any single technique.

Homoeopathy, with which this book is primarily concerned, has been known in the West for nearly two hundred years since Hahnemann made his astonishing researches into the action of potentized remedies. The principle *similia similibus curantur* — like is cured with like — is also expressed in the saying 'a hair of the dog that bit you'. Here, as in so many cases, a great truth is conveyed in a pithy sentence. The truth in question is that the power or potency of a remedy does not depend upon its quantity but upon its likeness to the cause of the disturbance. That which harms when taken in quantity, heals when administered in infinitesimal doses. The poison curare that instantly paralyses and kills animals and men, when separated from its material substratum will as rapidly heal a paralytic. The secret lies in separating the *pattern* of the remedy from its *material* base. This is Hahnemann's great discovery. The pattern is *potent*, whereas the material is *inert*. Potentizing is a very special and skilful operation which I believe must always be done by hand. It consists in blending the remedy with a neutral substance such as pure alcohol, water or sugar. Nine parts are discarded and one part is kept. This is repeated over and over again and each step adds one degree of potency. If the operation is performed six times, one part in a million remains and this is called *Potency Six*. The millionth part is far more positive in its action than the 999,999 parts that are thrown away. A potency of 30 means that only one part in 10^{30} remains. If we take the example of potentized common salt — *Nat. Mur.* — a single molecule weights 10^{-24} milligrams. It follows that a milligram of salt at a potency of 30 is not likely to contain even one molecule of the original material, and yet it can instantly stop a common cold, if it is taken the moment sneezing begins.

To those of us brought up to think in terms of measurable quantities of medicine in doses, rather than of remedies in potencies, it seems absurd to say that a remedy can work effectively when it is so diluted as to be virtually not there at all. This is, however, not so strange in the light of recent discoveries in the physical and biological science which have shown that a single quantum of electro-magnetic radiation, which is far smaller than an atom, can produce prodigious changes, such as inducing mutations in genes or exploding atom bombs.

An even better illustration of potency independent of quantity is given by the action of catalysts and enzymes. Chemical reactions differ in the ease and speed with which they occur. Some are very difficult and improbable. Most of those concerned with life are of this nature. A reaction that proceeds very slowly and with great difficulty can be accelerated and controlled by the presence of a catalyst that acts by its presence alone and does so often in very minute concentrations. This occurs because it is the pattern that acts and not the substance itself. It is the same with homoeopathy. As a remedy is potentized the substance is removed and the pattern is set free to act positively. This is why a very high potency is the most active.

Homoeopathy, which fifty years ago appeared strange and almost magical, fits into present day concepts of the physical universe and of life itself. Indeed, the study of homoeopathy has greatly helped me personally to understand better the connection between living and non-living matter. I write as one deeply interested in these questions: but I can hardly expect those who ask whether they should adopt homoeopathic medicine to make a scientific study of the theory of potentization.

Fortunately, the claims of homoeopathy do not depend upon theory, for they are reinforced by a hundred and eighty years of successful practice and by the experience of hundreds of thousands of people who owe their health and vigour to the right use of homoeopathic remedies. It is not hard to grasp the basis of natural medicine. Every physician, orthodox or unorthodox, agrees that the body is its own best healer. To act upon this marvellous organism from without by means of chemical agents can be a dangerous procedure and it often prevents the body from doing its own healing work.

I believe that in recent years physicians are becoming more sensitive to the danger associated with drugs of all kinds. A much more open attitude towards natural medicine is beginning to prevail. It is my personal conviction that the use of artificial remedies will diminish and doctors will turn more and more to natural remedies. The practitioner of natural medicine looks at the organism as a whole. He is concerned with health rather than disease, with 'healing' rather than 'curing'. He looks at symptoms, not in order to treat them, but to discern through them the hidden causes of the disturbance. Above all, he looks at the patient as a human being and is concerned with his entire body, soul and spirit.

It has become fashionable to talk of 'psychosomatic disorders' and to regard these as situated in a no-man's land in which neither physicians nor psychologists feel quite at home. There is a general tendency to disregard and neglect man's spiritual nature, that is his will, and yet the 'will to be healthy' is perhaps the most important factor in healing. 'Will' is very different from desire or from any impulse stemming from our emotional states. It is an act that comes from a sense of rightness and from awareness that each of us has a destiny to fulfil.

For this we must be healthy and vigorous and live long and strenuous lives. I have always been impressed in my dealings with Dr Sharma by his insistence upon the need for the 'will to be healthy'. The true natural healer can evoke this will in his patients because he is convinced that health and vigour are natural for man. He does not look upon his patients as 'suffering from disease' but as men and women in search of health. Health is harmony of body, soul and spirit, or body, feelings, mind and will. As the Greeks taught that the soul is a 'harmony', so does the practitioner of natural medicine seek to restore harmony to the whole of his patients. This is the principal reason why I believe that natural medicine is the healing science of the future.

This book makes the rudiments of natural medicine available to anyone who will read it carefully. Those who follow natural medicine are not passive guinea-pigs in the hands of their physicians, but active participants in the healing process. The more they know and understand how homoeopathic and other natural medicines work, the more they will benefit from the physician's care. I therefore recommend this book to all who realize that there is something lacking in the present-day 'orthodox' medicine.

I write as one who knows the difference and owes his present health and vigour to following natural medicine and accepting as a fundamental obligation to have the will to be strong and healthy in body, soul and spirit. For me this obligation is self-evident. It does not rest upon any system of belief or morality, but on the awareness that we possess a marvellous instrument which can give us unlimited satisfaction if we keep it in good order.

We are entering a most critical phase of human history. Life for the next fifty years will not be easy. We shall need to mobilize all our resources to get through successfully. Natural medicine has a great part to play in the great human venture.

INTRODUCTION

This handbook gives a brief introduction to the principles and practice of homoeopathy. If studied carefully it will enable the reader to look after his minor ailments and serve as an *aide-mémoire* in times of emergency. I hope that it will serve as a useful source of reference in your daily life.

In homoeopathy it is important that the patient should have some knowledge of what is an 'illness' and what is health; also of how a homoeopathic physician defines the function of a doctor, how I work and how I consider the patient should work with his doctor.

The patient should have a clear idea of how he should apply his thought to medicine and how, in practical life, he can learn to apply this to problems of health. Ultimately, the task of understanding lies with the patient. The means of understanding is the contract created between the patient and the doctor. This relationship may not change in principle, but will constantly change in practice.

Unorthodox and Orthodox Medicine

There is frequent dissension and heated debate between what is regarded as 'unorthodox medicine' and so-called 'orthodox medicine'. It should be made clear at the beginning that although there are certain principles upon which the two schools agree in theory, it is the attitude of mind *in practice* that is the main theme of variation between the orthodox and unorthodox. One might consider the division of the two schools as the difference between attitudes and practices more prevalent in the East and those found in the West.

In the East the art of treatment was, for many generations, in the hands of teachers. In the process of teaching about soul, spirit, psyche, chemistry, physics, biology and the like, they also taught of the effect of these on the body. The effect could either be for better or worse; when the effect was for worse, study of disease arose.

In the West doctors do not accept the responsibility of being a teacher. Without this broader concept, the Western approach is less able to treat *the man* suffering from an illness, and therefore most treat diseases of man without relating to him as a whole.

The basis of Western orthodox medicine is called allopathy. By definition, allopathy is 'the curing of a diseased action by inducing another action of a different or opposite kind'. The term derives from the Greek *alla* meaning 'different things' and *pathein* 'to suffer'. Even though we may not always be aware of it, the everyday application of allopathic principles is always with us. We can all diagnose a cold, even though the symptoms may vary considerably between one 'cold' and another; and most people have prescribed an aspirin for a headache, bicarbonate of soda for indigestion, and so on.

Homoeopathy, on the other hand, is much more closely related to the Eastern attitude towards man and his ills. The name comes from the Greek *homoia* meaning 'similar things' and again *pathein* meaning to 'to suffer'. Hippocrates stated: '. . . fever is produced by what it suppresses and is suppressed by what it produces'. Over a hundred years ago Hahnemann (1755-1843) proved the principle of curing by similars and thus became the father of modern homoeopathy.

It is a branch of medicine not very widely known in this country; even within the medical profession, few orthodox practitioners have made any thorough study of it. However, it should be noted that the homoeopathic physician has medical qualifications like all other physicians and is therefore conversant with the orthodox side of medicine. His homoeopathic qualifications are acquired in addition to those already achieved in orthodox medicine. This is not intended as any form of warranty or assurance but is a fact of the present circumstances.

In England, America and Europe, homoeopathy and other natural therapies are taught as post-graduate courses to an orthodox medical training. Under the present system a student is unable to make homoeopathy the basis of his medical training; he must first receive a training in orthodox medicine before he can study the unorthodox. In India the situation is quite different. It is possible for the student to qualify directly as a homoeopathic physician.

What has happened in India could easily happen here. The aims and objects of an ideal medical education, as laid down in an Indian government report in 1951, are worth stating in detail:

1. Physics, chemistry and biology should be of a high standard.
2. The teaching of physiology, anatomy and biochemistry — pre-clinical

subjects — should be completely re-orientated, and emphasis should be laid on the study of normal man with the following aims:

(a) To provide a basis for the understanding of the morphological, physiological and psychological principles which determine and influence the organization of the living body as a functioning unit.

(b) To relate and interpret the structural organization and normal physiology of the human body, and thus to provide the data on which to anticipate the disturbances of function which will probably result from interference with *normal structural relationships*.

(c) To enable the student to recognize the anatomical, physiological and psychological basis of the clinical signs and symptoms of disorder due to injury, disease, or mal-development and mal-chemistry.

(d) Similarly to help the student to understand the factors involved in the development of the pathological processes and the possible complications arising therefrom.

3. In the study of clinical subjects the purpose should be to teach the student the general principles of medicine; to train him to a sufficient degree of skill, to diagnose and treat common ailments and orientate his attitude towards medicine so that he sees his patient as a *whole*.

Orthodox medicine requires as essential the study of the basic sciences: chemistry, biology, physiology, biochemistry and anatomy. The latter half of the studies are concerned with the diagnosis and treatment of physical and psychological illness. The treatment rests upon a successful diagnosis of the illness. To this end, much specialized study and research has been done upon the single 'components' or 'units' that go to make up the human mechanism. Therefore, in orthodox medicine, disease and disease names have become the guiding measure of treatment and study and research mainly confined to the diagnosis of disease and to the effect of drugs on different organs and tissues.

In the field of research, tests are mainly carried out upon animals such as rabbits, mice, guinea-pigs etc. This is a bizarre deviation of research into human medicine. The anatomy, physiology, nerve structure and computer mechanisms, such as the autonomic nervous system, are totally different in animals from those of humans. Not even the bodily function of an anthropoid such as a gorilla is the same as that of man. Experiments are conducted on animals with various drugs and then transplanted, in theory, to man. To my mind this is erroneous and misguided research in the field of human medicine and is also a waste of considerable amounts of money and time.

In the field of homoeopathy it is the man suffering from disease who is, and has always been, the important focus; no effective treatment can begin without him first being studied as a *whole*. Homoeopathy studies the *patient* and his *individual* reaction to disease, and drugs, and seeks to provide a vital curative reaction within the person himself.

Thus it can be seen that the two schools are very different in their modes of practice. Any knowledge that you may have of orthodox medicine and its dosages is unlikely to be of much use to you in the homoeopathic treatment of your conditions and those of your family.

In the concentrated and exhaustive work that modern orthodox medicine has done in its study of the 'unit', the broader view has been lost of the effects of disease and of the therapeutic medicine or drug on the body as a whole. It is this difference in attitude that leads to the main distinction between orthodox and unorthodox medicine.

In turn, this style of practice is reflected in the transaction that takes place between the orthodox physician and the patient. The tacit agreement is that the physician should relieve the immediate situation and remove the inconvenience that the patient finds himself in on that particular day. Thus the illness is conceived as an imposition from an outside force (a hangover is caused by an excess of alcohol and *not* by my desire to drink); the patient demands nothing more than the removal of the imposition and to be allowed to return to his normal manner of living. Provided one understands that this is what the contract is, there should be no misunderstanding or disapproval of orthodox medicine. But, as a homoeopathic physician, I could not take part in such a contract. I function upon a different basis and the purpose of this book is to introduce the reader to these principles.

I do, however, believe that a wise homoeopath will try to keep abreast of new developments in orthodox medicine and in other branches of unorthodox medicine, so that he can make the best possible use of all the resources available for the benefit of the patients he is treating. In orthodox medicine, the study of units alone could ultimately lead to the study of the whole. For example, in the field of pathology, study has shown that, although a drug may have a beneficial effect on a single symptom, its broadcast effect can produce a gradual break-down of the processes of the body. Pathologists have found that the use of antibiotics (e.g. penicillin) destroys the bowel flora which absorb various vitamins and minerals. The result of this would be a deficiency disease such as ulcers in the mouth, diarrhoea, vomiting, loss of weight, and even depression and anxiety. In pathology this has created a shift in study born, not out of attitude, but out of necessity. One can only hope that many of the barriers and divisions that exist within the field of medicine will slowly break down in the interests of those people that it is pledged to serve.

Disquieted by the many side effects of drugs, the increased incidence of chronic disease and the lowering of general health standards, many people are seeking alternative methods of medicine. The science of homoeopathy has proved to be of great value to those who seek a more comprehensive and substantial insight into the causes of their disequilibrium. Many people are striving towards a greater understanding of themselves and their environment. This wish to know oneself as a whole is a concept of increasing importance in the evolution of modern man. Homoeopathy is a branch of medicine that wishes to serve and function by this concept.

PART ONE

THE ESSENTIALS OF HOMOEOPATHIC THERAPY

1

THE MAJOR PRINCIPLES
OF HOMOEOPATHY

There are two fundamental principles of medicine that all doctors accept, but which homoeopaths are more meticulous in carrying out.

The first is that the body contains repairing processes within itself, and that it is the physician's duty to make these processes active with the least possible medication.

The second principle is that in homoeopathy the physician always treats the patient *as a whole*, taking all signs and symptoms into consideration.

It is important to note that these two principles are closely inter-related. It is by the study of the patient as a whole that the physician will discover the means whereby he will be able to activate the repairing processes within the body. The way in which this happens, both for doctor and patient, will constantly change. The process continually develops from one cycle through to another. As a homoeopathic patient you will find it of great value to return to this book and re-read it in the light of your continuing progress.

Whether it is healthy or ill, each part of the body influences the body as a whole. Even though an illness may appear to be localized to a particular part of the body, the homoeopathic physician will always study the patient's condition as a whole before choosing his course of treatment. For example: the effect of a disease of the eye is not limited to the eye; various changes would occur in the rest of the body as a result of that disease. It would not only create changes in the blood supply, nerve fibre and general physiological structure of the eye, but would also create reactions to the disease in the rest of the body which would lead to further changes in the eye.

Therefore it is essential to know how the body as a whole has reacted to illness, and to see clearly the symptom pattern that the illness creates upon the healthy body. Each person, according to his constitution, will react individually to illness, will display a particular pattern of symptoms. It is by the careful study of this symptom pattern that the homoeopathic physician is able to choose the correct homoeopathic remedy.

It is essential that the homoeopathic physician has a wide general knowledge of how the body works. He must study the patient at all levels: not only his physical mechanisms, including the body's chemical processes, but also his mental and emotional characteristics, his inherited factors — culture, surroundings, family, genes, chromosomes, memories — and also his psyche and his spirit.

During treatment of a patient, the homoeopathic physician should aim to correct the patient's errors of thinking, movement, diet, etc., and, if necessary, refer him to relevant specialists. The patient is also studied in his environment, his home surroundings, and his work, in his world of weather, storms, cold, heat, rain and clouds. More mature and ancient sciences, such as the Chinese and the Ayurveda, put man further into the realm of atmospheric pressures, his planets and his relationship to the universe as a whole.

The individual exists within the universal structure; the single unit is the part of the whole. He or she is able to live within the universe either in a state of health or ill-health, in harmony or disequilibrium. Sometimes, as a result of living, the individual becomes ill and he will seek a cure. In other words, he seeks to return to the norm where there is no illness. If the illness is absent, the cure is not necessary; so a cure implies the necessity of living in such a way that illness does not occur.

This does not mean that one lives with the constant threat of being ill; on the whole, I think we tend to stabilize into health rather than remain on the precipice of ill-health. The quality of health is greater than the quality of disturbance. One need not worry about it being a continuous struggle.

So, we begin to see that a sickness is a process of understanding. This is not to say that I need to be sick in order to know, but rather if I do not know then I may become sick. There is no merit in ill-health — we should aim for healthy living which reduces its occurrence. One does not need a sickness to draw attention to the way one is living. It is the other way around; as a result of living I get a sickness which points out my difficulties in the experience. It is my belief that an illness is not something of which one need be afraid; rather it is an evolution, a self-representation of a human being at a stage at which something is demanded of him for the sake of experience. It is not an isolated event, but is invariably the result of the person's living as a whole.

When as a homoeopathic physician I meet a patient, I must decide the nature of my participation in this process. I must consider how much the patient is going to suffer. Is the inconvenience to his way of life going to be great or small and in what way can I help him live more peacefully and more lovingly within the world? Or alternatively, am I to ignore this broader, deeper spectrum and merely make the basis of my treatment the satisfaction of the patient's immediate demands and purposes? Am I instantly to curtail and prevent his experience of his illness?

Therefore, the patient's identification with the illness, as well as the behaviour of the illness to the patient, is a matter of mutual concern to the physician and the patient. Can I, the physician in the presence of the patient, share his experience; can I help him see a little more clearly whether the experience is essential for him or only an inconvenience from which he wishes to escape?

If, for instance, a patient comes to me with a cough, I, as the physician, have the privilege of wondering why he has chosen to have a cough, while the patient himself, in the condition in which he is, may well have lost that privilege. For him this is a stage of helplessness, of not knowing where to go. This helplessness can be relieved if I can indicate a programme for the patient to return to a state of health. This is the expression of the privilege; of knowing how a condition arose, and facing these facts in the present situation. This, I consider, is the essential relationship between the physician and the patient. If in the process of putting the cough right, I draw attention to the facts of how it happened, then it is possible to visualize how this would not happen.

If the sense is understood that an illness is not a super-imposed structure but a self-evolved understanding between the body and the mind, and between the physician and the patient, then we are going to approach the cure. As long as the patient does not think that it is the power of the doctor which will or will not cure the illness, but the power and the strength of the two together that will effect the cure, then I think an illness is a very simple process of understanding. If we can bear this in mind, then the *modus operandi* of the cure, or the receiving of the cure, is a matter of technical understanding.

So there is no short panacea to an illness. There is no particular way in which you eat, in which you sleep, in which you drink, in which you exercise, that is going to solve the problem. The problem is going to be solved by asking oneself: what is it all about? The constant posing of this question is fundamental to my concept of medicine.

I, as a physician, am simply a mirror you hold in front of yourself to see what has happened, and I, as a qualified person, interpret what you have not interpreted, put before you what I think is an ideal way of doing things, and then listen to you as to whether you will accept it or not. If you reject it, I will want to know why, so that I in my turn can study the matter again and find if there is an alternative viewpoint, or whether you rejected it to my satisfaction. If you have no intention of finding an alternative viewpoint, then to me, you are not my patient and I am not your physician.

I practise in the knowledge that, *essentially*, an illness is not a killing disorder, that death is not the ultimate of any illness, that death is an altogether different decision. The essence of an illness is your experience of that condition; a state of health is your own understanding of that day and that body. The contract between the physician and the patient is the study of this situation *as a whole*.

There is a third principle that is only accepted by homoeopathy from which, indeed, it takes its name (*homoia* — similar things). Homoeopathy uses medicine on the principle that there is nothing in nature that can harm which cannot also be used to cure, and that each thing can cure *only* what it causes or can cause.

Substances which are lethal poisons in large doses, in smaller doses tend to inhibit the functioning of the cells they affect, and in still smaller doses stimulate those cells to health. Dr Hahnemann, the founder of homoeopathy, studied this principle by administering certain drugs and medicines and following their effects on different levels of the human organism.

Each homoeopathic remedy has what is known as a symptom picture. Before a homoeopathic remedy can be used by a physician, it has to go through a series of '*provings*'. This is a complicated and meticulous process which was first used and developed by Dr Hahnemann. Very simply, this is the procedure: the remedy to be 'proved' is administered in specific doses at regular intervals to a group of *healthy* people of varying constitutions. All the symptoms that these people display, any deviation from the norm, are carefully recorded and tabulated by physicians and trained helpers. They record both psychological and physiological symptoms, starting with the vital organs of the body, then moving to the less important organs and from above downwards. The people under observation are kept in isolation, one from another, and therefore have no opportunities to compare symptoms. When this data has been collected it is then matched and tabulated until a clear overall picture or pattern of the remedy is produced.

In this way, Dr Hahnemann began to treat diseases by using remedies that produce the symptoms of a disease in a healthy person, in order to stimulate curatively the cells, tissues and organs which can be affected by those remedies.

So, it can be seen that drugs are sick-curing and sick-making: the sickness a drug produces is the one it cures. For example, belladonna can be used to cure scarlet fever because belladonna poisoning is 'so far as symptoms go' indistinguishable from those commonly produced by scarlet fever. Both cause the same burning skin, shining eyes and dilated pupils, dry, sore throat, and general excitement.

If, as a patient, you came to me with certain symptoms, I would then choose a remedy which in a healthy person produces the same picture. Thus homoeopathic remedies are given to suit individuals and their particular conditions, and are not directed at an illness: if bryonia, for example, is given for a cold, it does not follow that another patient will need bryonia when he has a cold, or even the same patient will need it when he has his next cold. So, there is no nice, convenient, particular remedy for anyone with catarrh, or with a cough, etc. The main aim of the homoeopathic remedy is to re-stimulate and return the vital force to its repairing function in the bodily processes. To arrive at a *correct* choice of remedy, one must constantly think in terms of the patient *as a whole*.

2
RECOGNITION OF THE STATES OF ILLNESS

Homoeopaths use the terms 'acute' and 'chronic' to distinguish between two different kinds of condition.

Acute Conditions
In an acute condition the body falters, but can regain balance if given time, protection and rest, and perhaps also the support of a homoeopathic remedy. Acute conditions are 'short and sharp'. For the homoeopathic doctor they are always different, although superficially repetitive. For instance, you may often have colds, but each cold will be different from the last, and so may need a different remedy. In acute conditions the body as a whole is not necessarily deteriorating; it may indeed be reacting and thus moving towards health.

Chronic Conditions
In a chronic condition, the body's vital force and reactive power have been disturbed to their depths; in homoeopathic language this is called miasm or miasmatic disorder. There will not usually be a spontaneous cure, unless a homoeopathic remedy is used to release the potentials of the recovering forces. Chronic conditions are always debilitating. They recur persistently, taking the same course each time (e.g. migraine, asthma, rheumatism). Their treatment should be left to the doctor. The layman should not attempt to prescribe remedies for chronic conditions as this needs medical understanding which embraces clinical as well as homoeopathic knowledge.

Symptoms and Recovery
It is a basic law of homoeopathy that recovery from a chronic condition proceeds:
1. from present conditions to past conditions,

2.   from above downwards,
3.   from inside to outside.

Symptoms displayed at any particular time by a patient undergoing homoeopathic treatment may be due to one aspect or another of the operation of this law. The patient will learn the validity of this law by observing the changes in himself and those around him in relationship to the prevailing environment.

It is also important to realize that many local phenomena, such as eruptions, discharges, and various aches and pains, are expressions of a deeper diseased condition; it is the condition, not those symptoms, which has to be cured. Treatment of the symptoms alone, and their suppression, would have harmful effects in the long run. Homoeopathic treatment attacks the underlying miasm, and for a short time may even cause an aggravation before bringing about a cure. A patient who does not know this might become alarmed and discontinue the treatment just at the moment when it was giving evidence of its effectiveness.

Homoeopathic remedies are not discontinued the moment you feel better; their action continues for a time after you stop taking them. In chronic conditions, the doctor will tell you when to stop taking the prescribed dose, as he will know the exact duration of the remedy's action.

Just as the homoeopathic doctor always treats the patient as a whole, taking *all* signs and symptoms into consideration, the same basic principle applies when you are treating yourself or one of your family for an acute condition. As you gradually gain experience, you will often be able to carry out the whole treatment yourself. In other cases you will know what to do before the doctor arrives, or how best to proceed if for any reason you cannot immediately get in touch with him. This handbook will give you guidance on when to call in a doctor, and also on the main things to look for before reporting to him when you have to do so. Clear, full and accurate reports on these occasions will save much time and anxiety all round.

3
THE PROCESS OF
DIAGNOSIS AND REMEDY

Having come this far with me, it is possible that you have discovered that your ideas are very different from mine. And, as a new patient, you may well ask how you can bridge this gap when you first come into my consulting room. Can you arrive with a new set of conceptions leaving your own preconceptions outside? Obviously you cannot.

Your preconceived ideas must come into the consulting room, must they not? They are part of your health and your ill-health, and you cannot leave your health outside the consulting room and only bring your ill-health.

To reiterate, my first consideration is always the contract I am going to undertake with you — what it is that you want of me and whether I am willing to come where you want me to go. If I find that as a physician or as a person I cannot come with you, then I would not do so. So, you have to deal with my preconceptions and conceptions and I have to deal with your preconceptions and conceptions as a prerequisite to such a contract.

Therefore, both doctor and patient need time in the consulting room to discuss such matters. Whenever I take on a new patient we always spend at least two hours together. During the first hour I decide what I am going to analyse about you and the second in finding how I can synthesize the analyses already made. Except in an emergency, I only take on a new patient when I can offer a total study. Thus, the average patient must be prepared to give this amount of time to see whether, together, we can form a group which can lead to health. If this is not done, we may prove mutually inadequate.

From this procedure I get to know the new patient and he begins to get to know me. It is also the basis upon which the process of general diagnosis and the correct selection of a remedy is able to grow.

When, in general day-to-day practice, I am trying to diagnose the patient's condition, I take into account only the deviation from the former healthy state of the individual which the patient himself feels, or those around him or the doctor observe. All these perceptible signs in a person indicate the whole extent of the disease, and together they form the only true picture in the condition.

As a doctor, I must have a thorough knowledge of the disease and its consequences, and of the patient's symptoms; I must know the powers of the medicine, and have the ability to select the particular remedy whose mode of action is most suitable to the case, also choose the exact quantity needed and its fitting period of repetition. Only then can I adapt the drug's healing virtue to the illness to be cured so that in most cases recovery will follow.

Whether an illness is physical, psychological or psychosomatic, a remedy which covers the whole disorder will always be sought. Homoeopathic treatment, therefore, does cater for psychological illnesses; especially those illnesses with a predominant psychological factor which are caused by changes in the body mechanisms (e.g. depression caused by a liver disorder or drunkenness). There can also be, of course, bodily changes of psychological origin, which, according to Rajinsky, are caused by 'ideas introduced to the mind'. Rajinsky suggests that: 'the "mind" works in very much the same way as the rest of the body, in a very fundamental way. Specifically, the mind treats ideas foreign to it just as the organism treats foreign bodies. It either rejects the idea or encapsulates it in order to preserve its integrity. An individual will reject any idea which is foreign to his experience in direct proportion to the degree of adjustment he will have to make in order to accept it.' (Because it may be of immediate inconvenience the mind fails to adapt a new attitude.) '. . . So, the individual often rejects ideas and suggestions that will be of help to him. Just as there are individuals who are more allergic than others, so there are people who are more emotionally allergic than others

NOTE: All practitioners will of course, on occasions, recommend common-sense treatment like rest, warmth, better diet, etc., but any non-homoeopathic medicines such as aspirin, tranquillizers, sleeping draughts and gargles can interfere with the action of homoeopathic remedies. It is also advisable to avoid deodorants and medicated cosmetics and soaps, dentifrice, ointments, face creams, toilet waters, bath salts, etc., especially any that contain camphor, menthol, hormones or mercury. (If in doubt whether preparations are medicated, play safe and do not use them.) Warning must also be given against the use of biochemic salts, with so-called homoeopathic potencies as part of their formula, because these would destroy the action of any homoeopathic remedy.

and who account for most of the psychosomatic disturbances. This principle implies that in order to teach a person something new it is necessary first to make him curious, so that what he chooses to accept and learn is not too foreign to him and so can be absorbed in relation to what he believes.'

BUILDING A SYMPTOM PICTURE
AND REPORTING TO THE DOCTOR

Before reporting any condition to the doctor, especially by telephone, try to marshal and write down as many of the following facts as you can. This will help give the doctor a clear picture of the patient as a whole and can enable him to advise more quickly.

1. Temperature.
2. Pulse.
3. Variations in environment and behaviour.
4. Inputs: what is being put into the body.
5. Outputs: all exertions and excretions.
6. Any instructions being currently followed, especially any remedies being taken, and whether in the form of powder or pills.

1. Temperature
This may be taken by mouth, rectum, in the groin or in the armpits. With small children it is safest to take it rectally or in the groin. The rectal temperature is roughly 0.4°C (1.4°F) above the oral, which is slightly higher than the axiliary and groin temperature. When reporting, state where it was taken and at what time. It will be lower in the middle of the night and in the morning, higher in the afternoon and late evening. Evaporating sweat can bring the temperature down.

The thermometer should be registered for at least four minutes. It will not rise beyond that time and in any shorter period the temperature may not be recorded accurately. The range of normal temperatures varies greatly with different people, from 36°C to 37.2°C (96.8°F to 99°F). It is helpful if you know your normal temperature. To find this out, you should take it several times a day for three days when in normal health.

To many people the word temperature is synonymous with fever. But I would stress again that the word temperature is not synonymous with fever, so don't say 'I haven't got a temperature' or assume it is normal without having taken it. There is, in fact, no struggle in the body which does not produce a temperature reaction. If the temperature goes up, the body is making an effort to cure the illness. If the temperature goes down, either the body has coped with the situation or it is giving up the struggle.

2. Pulse
A normal pulse ranges from 70 to 90 beats per minute. What you have been doing or feeling may have considerable effect on the pulse rate, and if it is more or less than normal, you should note any such circumstances.

3. Variations in Environment and Behaviour
Note the conditions and variations of the environment; are you in the town, country, indoors, outdoors; is it dry, wet, windy, humid, etc.? The emotional environment of the patient should also be noted.

Also note the conditions and variations in the body (physical symptoms): headaches, pains, sweat, swelling, stiffness, feeling too hot or too cold, etc.

The patient's behaviour should also be observed (mental symptoms): anxiety, apathy, anger, appetites, cravings and aversions, dreams (pleasant and unpleasant), etc.

4. Inputs
Inputs means *all* the things that are taken into the body. This includes the air we breathe as it contains pollens, chemicals and traces of elements. If, for example, one was by the sea, the air would contain degrees of sodium, ozone and chlorides. Also in this category are solids and liquids taken by mouth, smoking, inhalations, drugs, embrocations, injections and so on.

5. Outputs
Outputs means all things that move from the *inside* of the body to the outside. This includes physical and mental exertion, and all excretions:
(a) Stools.
(b) Vomiting.
(c) Urine.
(d) Sweat.
(e) Discharges from apertures of the body, like nasal, rectal, vaginal discharges, phlegm from coughs etc.

(f) The stage of the menstrual cycle and symptoms before, during, and after menses.

With all excretions note frequency, colour, consistency, contents.

Always try to work in a systematic and orderly way. As a guiding principle always assess the patient's symptoms by working from above downwards; starting with the head, eyes, ears, nose, throat, chest and so on down to the feet.

By following the other guiding principles mentioned above, the patient and his illness can then be placed within the broader context of the whole.

Building a Symptom Picture

When looking after anyone who is ill, do not try to gain too much information from the patient concerned. Information gained from your observation is generally of greater value. When taking notes of a case, either for a report to the doctor, or else to enable you to choose a remedy for treatment at home, it is helpful to bear in mind the following points:

1. Your own careful observation of the patient is of vital importance. Therefore, always try to avoid questions that suggest certain answers.

    For example: Not — have you got a headache? but rather — do you have any pain? Not — does it hurt when you move? but rather — is it better or worse by movement?

2. Do not ask questions which may be answered by a direct affirmation or negative.

    For example: instead of asking 'are you hot?' look around, observe, and find whether the patient is overcovered or not covered, and ask whether he would like another blanket, or the window open, etc.

3. Never ask alternative questions, such as 'If you don't like tea, would you prefer coffee?' or 'If you don't like hot drinks, do you like ice cold drinks?'

4. Confine yourself to one symptom at a time.

5. Never ask questions along the line of a remedy, i.e. while reading remedy symptoms.

    As Herring, a well-known authority on homoeopathy, said: 'Measure the head and then the hat, not the hat and then the head.'

When taking notes of a case, it is important to avoid bias and pre-judgement. Prepare your case with an open mind, and do not look up colds and coughs because you have decided the patient is suffering from one. An accurate choice of treatment of the patient can be arrived at by the creation of a complete picture.

When offering the doctor a daily report of the patient's progress, always try to begin with how you consider the patient to be, in himself, as a whole. And, remember, the patient is the person who is most likely to express an opinion as to his general condition, so let him express it. 'How are you in yourself?' is always a key question. From the basic question one can proceed to a detailed enquiry in the manner already indicated. The sum total of the detail information is as important as the patient's reply to the question 'How are you in yourself?'

5

HOMOEOPATHIC REMEDIES

A homoeopathic remedy is available in four forms: mother tincture form, pillules, globules and triturations.

Mother tinctures. These are extracts of original substances or remedies prepared according to regulations laid down by Hahnemann, mostly in strong alcohol.

Pillules. These are made of pure cane sugar able to absorb potentized remedies prepared in alcohol. A few drops of alcohol potency are put on to the pillules for absorption. They are easily handled, and if kept in a well-corked bottle will retain their virtue for many years. They are very suitable for domestic use, especially for the beginner.

Globules, about the size of poppy seeds, are prepared in the same manner as pillules, and are very convenient for administering to infants. They are not very easily handled, and their appearance has done much to cause ridicule and prejudice.

Triturations are in the form of powder, or tablets made from powder, containing a portion of the original drug triturated with a given quantity of sugar of milk. They are necessary for administering the lower attenuation of insoluble medicines, such as *Carbo veg.*

Drops and pillules are easily divided into any number of doses by mixing them with the corresponding number of spoonfuls of water, and giving one spoonful for a dose.

Pillules and globules may be taken dry on the tongue or sucked, but should not be swallowed whole; it is best to dissolve them in the mouth slowly. They may, however, be dissolved in pure soft water.

Triturations (powders) should always be taken dry on the tongue.

Using and Choosing a Remedy

Do not be in too much of a hurry to use a remedy for an acute condition. For one thing, you may get rid of it by simple things like warmth, rest, drinks, particular foods. Secondly, the condition is an index of a struggle between the processes of the illness and the repairing processes of the body. The body may sometimes have to produce a cold, for instance, in order to eliminate toxins and thus regain health. Therefore you need only intervene with a remedy if the repairing processes are losing the battle. This applies also to symptoms like fever (high temperature) and pain.

Fever should not be considered an enemy. It shows that the body is already making a definite defensive effort towards curing the illness. A great deal of comfort can be brought by rest, cold compresses, cold and refreshing drinks, fresh air and exclusion of draughts. If, despite these things and any remedy you use, the fever continues, you should consult the doctor.

Pain is nature's signal pointing to a disorder or the need for repair. A homoeopathic remedy is not called for if you can bring relief by simple measures, e.g. applying hot water bottles to a stomach-ache, ice to bruises, kaolin poultices to abscesses, vinegar and water to headaches. But if the pain persists or grows worse, so that you feel a special remedy is necessary, then you want one which will deal with the cause of the pain. Never use something like aspirin to counteract the pain itself, for you would be masking the cause, which would only lead to more complications and perhaps worse pain in the future.

To repeat: never treat symptoms in isolation. Before you choose a remedy in a given case, you should find at least three major symptoms of that remedy, and preferably four (or more). If one of your children is unwell, listen to and observe all the symptoms, do not look for a remedy too soon, but wait for the full picture to show itself.

Here is an example: Jane comes home from school looking pale. She says she has a headache, and she doesn't want her evening meal. Her temperature is 98.4°F. Put her to bed, give her plenty of lemon and honey, and after a night's sleep she may be better. If she is not, she may have a fever and a streaming cold, or a sub-normal temperature with vomiting and diarrhoea. Now is the time to choose a remedy, carefully matching symptoms with remedy.

Each member of the family who begins to be unwell should be

considered as an individual, with a remedy chosen accordingly. Because a remedy cured Father's cold, it will not necessarily cure John's.

When suffering from a condition yourself, you may find it hard to see your own symptoms objectively and in the right perspective. Where practical, therefore, it is worth asking a 'homoeopathic' friend or relative to evaluate the symptoms and choose a remedy.

Do not try to treat acute conditions in friends and neighbours who go to a different doctor — you do not know enough about their constitutions. If you give a friend a dose of *phosphorus*, say, for a bad cough, and phosphorus happens to be his constitutional remedy, you will take him through the gamut of a whole reactive force which will confuse his doctor and not help him. *Your* coughs and colds are different from his.

Remedy Epidemicus is a remedy which I and some homoeopathic colleagues may have discovered on getting the same symptom picture from a number of patients at a given time. If you find you are suffering from the same symptoms as several people round you, you should contact the surgery to see whether there is a remedy epidemicus: but do not rely on it being the same remedy for two epidemics. Similarly, there are remedies which are effective with many people in particular climatic conditions: e.g. *Aconite*, *Bryonia* or *Nux vomica* when there are cold dry winds; and *Natrum sulph.* or *Rhus tox.*, in a sudden cold, wet spell.

There is no such thing as a prophylactic use of an acute remedy, e.g., to prevent colds if you know you are subject to them, or to stop a hangover coming if you know you are likely to drink too much on a particular occasion. The condition must arise before it can be relieved. Homoeopathy as preventive medicine is very complex, and should be left to the doctor — except, of course, that you can prevent many ailments by common sense, by eating and drinking the right things, getting enough rest, etc.

For good reasons the doctor will usually not tell you the name of your constitutional remedy or of a remedy he is giving you for a chronic condition. But he will naturally tell you the name of the acute remedy he advises and this will educate you in choosing remedies for the future. Before you feel confident enough to decide for yourself, you can always ask him whether a remedy you have chosen is correct. If you find your choice is not right, do not be discouraged, for you will gradually learn by experience and develop something like an instinct for the right remedy. But whether the remedy has been chosen for you or you have chosen it yourself, always keep a careful record of what it is, the potency, frequency and quantity, and the symptoms which called for it.

If you think you have used the wrong remedy, because the acute condition is persisting, you should refer the matter to the doctor. Homoeopathic remedies will never do harm in the way that allopathic drugs often do; but if used in the wrong place, they will mask the condition, and so will confuse the doctor about your general state of health and your remedy.

When using a remedy for an acute condition or an injury, you should discontinue all previous homoeopathic remedies prescribed until you have consulted the doctor; but you can go on taking any vitamin tablets, etc. that may have been prescribed.

Potency, Frequency and Quantity

In determining these factors, you should consider the patient's age, sex and habits as well as the nature of the disease. The cleanliness and state of the mouth must also be considered, as it is here that the main absorption takes place. Before taking any remedy the mouth should be rinsed with water.

The potency of a remedy will not greatly concern you at the initial stage, since the home chest should only contain remedies of potency 6 and/or 12.

If you are certain that the remedy you select is the correct one, start with potency 12; otherwise use potency 6. If the latter does not act, try another indicated remedy at potency 12. Similarly, if the remedy at potency 6 works but the condition recurs after a few days, use the same remedy at potency 12.

The frequency depends on the severity of the attack. With severe and frequent vomiting and diarrhoea, you may need to take the remedy every fifteen minutes, but the frequency should be reduced at the first signs of improvement to perhaps half hourly, hourly, and so on. In milder cases, you may start with two pills every two hours, reducing it to two every three hours, then every four hours, and gradually tail it off over a period of three days. (Always tail off a homoeopathic remedy; if you end it abruptly, you may get a remedy reaction.)

The correct quantity of a remedy will normally be two pills. When, however, there is a very 'foul' mouth (after a hangover, for instance, or heavy smoking), that is a sign that two pills will not be enough. You will need four or even eight at a time to give the remedy a chance of better absorption.

Usually, the desirable times for taking remedies are on rising in the morning and/or at bedtime. If prescribed more often, they may be taken an hour before a meal or two hours after. Nothing should be 'taken' by mouth (which includes smoking and teeth-cleaning), for twenty minutes before or after; or ten minutes before or after, when the remedy is taken more frequently, as in acute conditions. In no circumstances should a patient be woken from sleep to take a remedy.

Buying and Keeping of Remedies

You should obtain your homoeopathic remedies only from reliable sources, such as homoeopathic chemists, who know the value of potency and how easily these remedies can be destroyed: therefore they make sure the remedies are not kept in a window exposed to strong sunlight, nor polluted by fumes, perfumes, etc., nor stored near drugs, chemicals or other medicines.

If properly kept, your remedies will last a life-time. Never use the stock-bottle for dispensing a remedy. Take a few pills out of the bottle, put them in a clean envelope, then put the bottle away again. If a container is broken, the remedy can be transferred to a new clean envelope; but if pollution is suspected, it is advisable to obtain a fresh supply of the remedy.

Remedies kept in snuff-boxes, or carried with scent and powder in handbags, or put in the same pocket as cigarettes and matches without enough covering and protection, tend to lose their efficacy.

Do not label the remedies 'Belladonna for diarrhoea', etc. It is the whole symptom picture, not the name of an illness or complaint, which will decide the remedy you use.

Home Chest

Your home medicine chest should be kept out of the reach of children and away from strong light or smells. It should contain the following remedies in pill form, potency 6 and 12.

Aconite	Calcarea carbonica
Allium cepa	Calcarea phosphorica
Apis mellifica	Calendula officinalis
Argentum nitricum	Carbo vegetabilis
Arnica	Causticum
Arsenicum album	Chamomilla
Belladonna	Chelidonium
Bryonia	Dioscorea villosa

Drosera
Eupatorium
Ferrum phosphoricum
Gelsemium
Hepar sulphuris calcareum
Hypericum
Ignatia
Kali bichromicum
Kali carbonicum
Kali phosphoricum
Magnesia phosphorica
Mercurius

Natrum muriaticum
Natrum sulphuricum
Nux vomica
Phosphorus
Pulsatilla
Pyrogenium
Rhus toxicodendron
Ruta graveolens
Silica
Spongia tosta
Staphysagria
Urtica urens

also:

Ascorbic Acid tablets 50mg and 1g.
Vitamin B$_1$ tablets.
A.C.U. ointment (equal portions of *Arnica*, *Calendula* and *Urtica urens* prepared in either a greasy or non-greasy base).
A.C.U. lotion.
Golden Eye ointment.
Verbascum ear oil (a preparation of Verbascum oil with glycerine).
Castor oil (for removing foreign bodies in the eyes).
Kaolin.
Hamamelis (Witch Hazel).
Glycerine suppositories (adult and child size).
Various bandages (including crepe and triangular).
Elastoplast (unmedicated, with and without pads).
Safety pins, scissors, tweezers, cotton wool, gauze, sticks for swabs, optule.
Notebook and pencil for recording symptoms and remedies.
Lemons, honey, glucose, cider vinegar, rose-hip syrup, charcoal biscuits and arrowroot, should always be kept in the house.

PART TWO

DAILY LIFE FOR THE WHOLE PERSON

6

HYGIENE, VACCINATION AND IMMUNIZATION

Hygiene is that branch of science concerned with preserving health, and preventing disease by the removal of pollution caused by man and society. Improved conditions, brought about by modern technology have been vital factors in promoting hygiene and so maintaining better health. Improved hygiene has perhaps caused more changes in general health than any other aspect of modern science; various illnesses and disorders have become less rampant, and in many cases have been almost or completely wiped out. The standard of hygiene that we have so far achieved has been built up by many years of effort. But the situation is anything but perfect; through misuse of our resources we have a new form of pollution more serious in its consequences than previous forms of pollution.

For the individual, the essence of hygiene is the working towards a better, more harmonious balance of the mind and body as a whole. It is in the context of this endeavour that the individual begins to see himself in relationship to the family, the community and the world at large. This is the measure of true progress. The degree to which modern man has failed to discover his relationship to the world in which he lives, his lack of interest and concern, is reflected in the frightening quantity of pollution that we are now spreading across the planet.

For the individual to solve his own immediate problem of pollution may well not be a genuine solution as his actions will not necessarily decrease the quantity of pollution for the community at large. If the community suffers because of its lack of hygiene then, in return, the individual will ultimately also suffer, for he is part of the community.

No arguments of insufficient finance can excuse our failure to live in harmony with the world into which we are born. We have both the finance and the resources, so that cannot be the problem. A solid basis has been established for promoting a high standard of general health; but, in order to achieve this aim, I believe that we have to consider more carefully the way in which we view the world and use the resources that we now have at our disposal.

Vaccinations and Immunizations

The question of vaccinations and immunization is a difficult one, but there is much evidence that these are harmful to the system. I believe that the use of vaccines ignores the individual's improved hygienic standards. By relying on the antibodies that the vaccine creates, the body's repairing processes are thrown into disuse so that the natural defence mechanism no longer works. Illness such as measles, chicken pox, mumps and scarlet fever alert the body's defences and produce the ability to withstand viral and other infections in later life.

At birth one has certain hereditary susceptibilities and immunities. It is my belief that research should be directed to find these 'failures of memory' and 'successful memory' in genesis — in our D.N.A. Immunizations, therefore, should be aimed at the specific 'failure of memory'.

Dr Michael Lane and J. Donald Miller in a 'Reconsideration of Continued Childhood Vaccinations Against Smallpox' produced a very brief, excellent résumé of the problem at the sixth Annual Immunization Conference, March 1969, in Atlanta, Georgia. They state that there are each year at least seven deaths attributed to vaccines and that the figures may well be under reported. The present risks of vaccination are thereby understated and the many after effects, such as morbidity due to vaccinia, are ignored. I believe it is important that statistics reporting complications and resultant illnesses such as asthma, warts, growths, skin rashes, encephalitis, etc. should be compiled.

No imported cases of smallpox have occurred in the U.S.A. for 30 years; 47 imported cases occurred in Western Europe (population 700,000,000) of which 30 caused further cases. This resulted in a total of 723 cases of which 111 resulted in death.

The U.S.A. vaccination programme showed, in its 30 years operation, that 210 deaths were due to vaccination only.

Conyberte and Wynn Griffiths from Great Britain found 2.8 deaths per million primary vaccines. No child primary vaccination figures have been provided.

Lane and Miller state that the current claims of the effectiveness of complete protection of the population by vaccination are overstressed, and that, depending upon the country, between 10-15 per cent of the population is not protected. Also, the risks of importation are, in fact, close to zero.

Even from an orthodox viewpoint, no sound case can be made out for mass immunization, and early childhood vaccination cannot be justified. Also, if adult vaccination programmes are kept to an absolute minimum, there will be no risk of spread of death.

The unorthodox view is that hygiene, cleanliness and the isolation of cases have brought about the changes in world statistics. This is also felt to be the case with diseases such as diphtheria, scarlet fever, whooping cough and complications caused by these illnesses.

The case for poliomyelitis immunization also fails statistically because complications and the resultant loss of muscle power caused by polio immunizations make it futile to depend upon a programme of immunization rather than a programme of teaching hygiene and cleanliness. The need, above all, is for a programme of tests for natural immunity against these illnesses.

B.C.G. vaccine (tuberculosis) and its routine use has also brought a great many complications. The aim should be to test children, as we do now, and when they show failure of immunity they should be closely watched, tested and *perhaps* x-rayed at intervals. This should be done rather than introduce B.C.G. vaccine and then discover a high susceptibility to a vaccine causing a severe tuberculosis, tubercular encephalitis or other well known complications.

Some of the vaccinations and immunizations which travellers undergo before visiting certain countries are legally compulsory, and others are not compulsory but are considered advisable.

In both cases you should consult the physician: in the former so that he can clear the harmful effect from the system afterwards; in the latter to discuss the pros and cons of undergoing them at all.

He may in fact decide that you are exempt because it would be grossly harmful to your health. Changes in attitude about routine need for vaccination under the studied guidance of World Health Organization are under way and it is now not compulsory to be vaccinated except in cases where you are travelling from an endemic area. See *The Truth About Vaccination and Immunisation* by Lily Loat (Health for All Publishing Company, 17-18 Henrietta St., London WC2).

7

CARE OF THE BODY

The clothing one wears has an important effect on health. Avoid wearing nylon and other man-made fibres (except rayon), especially when they come into direct contact with the skin, since they prevent aereation and insulate the body from its environment, even when holes are left in the fabric. It is best not to wear tight clothes, especially such things as corsets.

Skin and Hair

Skin is a functional organ. It has vestiges of a breathing apparatus, and is in fact a third kidney, since the composition of sweat and urine are similar. The skin helps to protect the body surface, prevents oozing of fluids from the body, stores vitamins (especially vitamin D), eliminates acids that are not dealt with by the kidneys, and so aids the kidney function. It is also an absorptive area, since anything applied to the skin gets absorbed. It is very important to bear this in mind when using cosmetics, embrocations, bath preparations, etc. and before sunbathing, having ultra-violet ray treatment, etc.

Any recurrent irritation, eczema, rash, large burn or wound should be brought to the physician, rather than treated at home. Suppressing skin disorders can have dire consequences.

In the use of towels, face cloths and other items of personal hygiene, it is important to know the individuality of skin. The flora of the skin varies and can be transplanted on to other skins and be harmful. Besides this, active skin disorders like acne, impetigo, scabies etc., have to be kept in mind.

Remember that in the understanding and care of the skin, you should include the scalp, which is a thicker skin than the rest but more generously supplied with blood.

Dandruff is a major medical problem, fairly resistant to treatment, about which you should consult your doctor. Some hair preparations can result in suppressive illnesses, because although they treat the dandruff locally they may actually damage the scalp or contain drugs which can do harm to the system generally. Many people do not take this matter seriously, and these include rash physicians!

Lemon juice can be helpful in mild cases of dandruff. Cut a lemon in half and rub both halves briskly into the scalp. Allow juice to remain for ten minutes and then wash out with plenty of water. Another similar wash can be made with sour milk. Try one or the other over a period and note which one suits your needs.

Care of the Eyes
It is important to learn to use the eyes in an easy and relaxed manner. Otherwise tensions may occur which can impair good vision and cause other problems. There is normally no need for eye-baths and eye-washes in the care of the eyes, except for using clean water, as below.

Splashing the Eyes with Water
This should become a regular habit. Every morning splash your eyes twenty times with hot water, then twenty times with cold. Repeat last thing at night, but starting with cold and ending with hot. The eyes must be closed, the head bent over a basin, the water splashed on the eyelids.

Palming
A useful exercise whenever the eyes are tired or aching, and could well be done once a day. Sit with your elbows on a table, close your eyes, and place them in the palms of your hands. The head should rest lightly on the hands, with the fingers crossed over on the forehead. Now forget your eyes and think about some pleasant experience, a beautiful view, lovely music or poetry, anything that makes the mind relax. There is no special length of time for doing this, even two or three minutes will help.

Near and Far-focusing
A great help for both short- and far-sighted people, and should be done without glasses.

The short-sighted should focus on to something near, then on to something in the distance, trying to pick out particular colours or shapes. Repeat many times. Although the things in the distance may appear blurred, it will help to stop the eyes becoming fixed and tense, which can often cause a headache or feeling of 'sand-in-the-eyes'.

The far-sighted should do the same exercise, but concentrate on seeing things as near to the eyes as possible, like looking at very small print, or bringing a book to within six inches of their eyes. It does not matter if they cannot actually see the letters; the important thing is the quick adjustment of the eye muscles.

Bates eye exercises are of great value in all eye conditions, and a Bates Practitioner's opinion is often extremely helpful. Unfortunately there are very few in England, but for further information please refer to The Secretary, The Bates Association, 49 Queen Anne Street, London W1.

Foreign Body in the Eye

Do not remove anything from the eye unless it is big and easy to get out. If there is a foreign body in the left eye, rub the right eye, and vice versa, as the movement of the eyeballs synchronize, and this will help the particle to come out. If it does not come out, then put one drop of castor oil in each eye, and the particle should float out quite easily. A single oral dose of *Aconite* 200 can remove foreign bodies from the eyes.

Some indicated remedies — *Aconite, Staphysagria.*

Styes

Styes are small boils on the eyelids. Do not squeeze or try to puncture them, as this will only drive the infection deeper. Apply warm, wet compresses soaked in A.C.U. lotion (one teaspoonful to a pint of water) several times a day. Warm water that has been boiled will do if A.C.U. is not available. When the stye breaks, just wipe away the pus with a pad soaked in the lotion.

If you get many styes, you should consult your doctor.

Some indicated remedies — *Aconite, Hepar sulph., Pulsatilla, Staphysagria.*

Care of the Ears

Careful and regular cleansing of the ears as far as the little finger can go with a covering of soft gauze or lint will help to keep them free from wax. In later age the hair growth very often attracts dirt and holds it, the hair may break and the ear can get blocked. This can be cleared and wax removed by filling the ear with hydrogen peroxide, letting it bubble and then run out. If the wax is badly impacted and not cleared by repeatedly using this method, it is best to leave it for the attention of the doctor.

It is important when travelling, particularly by air, to see that the eustachian tubes do not get blocked. This can easily happen if you have a cold, cough or catarrh at the time. Gargling with A.C.U. lotion (teaspoonful to a pint) before you start and chewing gum during the journey will help to keep the tubes free. On no account should you blow your nose very hard in conditions of pressure.

Earache which is caused by colds and coughs is better treated by attending to the cause, though inhalations and drops of Verbascum oil can be helpful.

About a third of the cases of earache in children are due to teething, so think in the same terms as you would to relieve toothache. A hot water bottle on the ear, and warm Verbascum oil may be used.

Indicated remedies — *Aconite, Arnica, Hypericum, Pulsatilla, Hamamelis* (Witch Hazel).

Care of the Teeth

The functions of the teeth are very important. They exercise a large influence in the production of articulate sounds, and have a keen sense of touch by which they recognize the texture of food and can detect the presence of a foreign body in the mouth. Their most important function is, of course, mastication, by which food is prepared with the aid of the saliva, for the essential preliminaries to digestion. The loss of teeth in many animals is often the limit of their life. In human beings, however, exercising the teeth is a very important need. The more hard and alive the food eaten, the better the teeth will be. The failure of proper mastication ending in badly chewed morsels is a frequent cause of severe dyspepsia.

The condition of the teeth ought to be of great interest to the physician. The pathology of teeth should draw his attention to their interaction with the digestive system. Nervousness in eating, or fast eating, and inefficient mastication can cause digestive and other maladies.

Gums, jaws and teeth are all closely connected, and in many cases the teeth are the starting point of disease in other structures. The portion of the mucous membrane of the mouth which covers the gums is modified to a certain extent, in that here it becomes incorporated and attached to the periostium of the bone to form a muco-periostium, and therefore severe dental decay can implicate the jaw and the surrounding structures. Troubles like gingivitis and inflammation of the gums are frequently accompanied by general digestive troubles, and are often the results of dirty or septic teeth, though equally they may be repercussions of digestive troubles.

I would emphasize the necessity and the virtues of saliva on the gums and mouth, for it contains chemical substances which are vital both for its healing qualities and for keeping the mouth healthy. I have yet to find severe dental disorder in a person who allows the action of the saliva to follow its natural course.

Time and again you find people who smoke or have a 'nightcap' just before going to bed. It is during the six or seven hours of sleep that the saliva can play its full part in cleansing and healing the mouth, gums and teeth. To pollute the saliva just before the mouth has its longest period of rest means that you are not giving it the full opportunity to function as nature intended it should.

It is equally important that during the day the chemical properties of the saliva should be given an opportunity to work. Many people give their mouths no respite at all, they are either smoking, having a cup of tea or a glass of sherry, and then it is time for a meal, followed perhaps by chocolates or sweets, and then more cigarettes. Though they may be prepared to clean their teeth with a tooth brush twice a day, their mouths would be far healthier if they gave them a rest, and let the saliva do its work.

This constant use of the mouth, entailing no salivary action, is one of the most difficult problems for the physician to overcome; the patient very often needs a severe reprimand or even a psychologist! It ought to be pointed out to the sufferer from bad teeth, gums and mouth, that unless he gives his mouth a rest so that the saliva can function properly, there can be very little chance of his condition improving, let alone being cured.

In the care of teeth it is important to keep them free from all particles of food which might get lodged in between them; also when cleaning them use as much water as possible. The best way of cleaning the teeth is to rinse water through the gaps by the means of forceful gargling and swilling. It is good practice to do this several times per day. An excellent way to keep the gums healthy is to massage them, both upper and lower, inside and out, with the forefinger, for at least a minute. Please note that cleaning the surface of the tongue each morning is also important.

Recently I have suggested to very heavy smokers that they should use chewing gum, with very good results on the teeth and the general health of the mouth.

As far as possible, use unmedicated tooth-paste. Recent research has proved that the best way for non-vegetarian people to prevent decay is to eat an apple after cleaning their teeth.

If a gargle or mouthwash is needed on account of dental treatment, use hydrogen peroxide, or A.C.U. lotion, diluted one teaspoonful to two pints of water. Both these will help the healing process and alleviate bruising pains.

Patients should be warned that certain dentifrices containing potencies of sulphur or other ingredients are harmful to remedies given orally.

Your dentist should be told that you are homoeopathically treated. In my experience injections and gas for tooth extractions have very little effect on the system. But if the dentist advises oral medication afterwards, or there is a question of treating pain after extractions, it is advisable to ask him to inform the physician.

Toothache

Try common-sense treatment like applying ice or hot water to the place where the ache is. But when the tooth is extremely sensitive to anything cold, the pain is probably caused by a nerve. If you are undergoing dental treatment you will probably know the cause of the pain, and the dentist will have advised you on what action to take.

Toothache can be helped by chamomile tea.

Teething Troubles in Children

These are mostly accommodative struggles. The body as a whole is trying to provide the minerals necessary for forming teeth, while the mouth and gums are getting used to having teeth in them.

A great deal of patience is needed at this stage. The child should have a hard teething ring to bite on, made of smooth ivory, bone, or even silver if you cannot afford gold! (but not plastic).

Chamomile tea will reduce pain.

Indicated remedies — *Arnica, Belladonna, Hypericum, Chamomilla, Pulsatilla, Mag. carb., Mag. phos.*

Care of the Feet

It is important to go bare-foot as often as possible and I advise patients not to put their children into shoes at an early age and in any case not before they can walk properly. When buying shoes make sure they are not too tight and it is best to choose leather soles. High heels are a scourge to a woman's pelvis but have become inevitable in society today; they should be worn as little as possible and casual footwear should be encouraged.

Stockings and socks should ideally be made of cotton, wool, silk or rayon, and I attribute many diseases, such as varicose veins, athlete's foot and dropped arches, to the use of man-made fibres like nylon and terylene, which unfortunately seems almost universal.

Bunions, corns, warts and fallen arches are caused by never going about with bare feet, wearing high heels, rubber soles, etc. When going to a chiropodist it is essential to tell him that you are treated homoeopathically and do not believe in the use of ointments, creams and applications which are likely to be absorbed into the system through the skin.

Sprains and tired feet are best treated by putting the feet in hot water containing one teaspoonful of A.C.U. lotion to one pint.

Athlete's Foot
This is a condition caused by a fungal growth often in the web of the toes and, like eczema, can be a constitutional condition; therefore medical advice should be sought. The fungus does not grow except in the presence of moisture, therefore after washing feet surgical spirit should be used to keep the web dry. Simple dusting powders like Fullers Earth may be used, but do not use medicated powders.

Indicated remedy — *Silica.*

Ingrowing Toenails
These are nearly always caused by bad footwear. When cutting the nail make a small V-shaped cut in the centre, which will release the pressure from the sides of the toe. Pure lambswool drawn under the sides of the nail will prevent deep growth into the nail bed.

Poultices and Inhalations
Poultices are most useful for minor or small abscesses, and for suppurating places, on account of the moisture they convey, and can be applied when the skin or the underlying structure is inflamed. They reduce the pain by relaxing tension and promoting perspiration. Poultices can be made in the following ways and wrapped in gauze before application.

Linseed Meal Poultice. Pour boiling water into a heated bowl, and sprinkle the meal into this while stirring the mixture, until a thin smooth dough is formed.

Bread Poultice. Put slices of bread in a basin, pour boiling water over them and place by the fire for a few minutes. Pour off the water and replace by fresh boiling water. Pour this off again and mash the bread with a fork to form a poultice. This type of poultice is valuable for its bland non-irritating properties.

Carrot Poultice. Boil carrots until soft, mash with a fork and apply in the ordinary way. They are said to make wounds cleaner and healthier.

The water and vessels used when making a poultice must be absolutely clean.

A dry fomentation may be used when heat alone is required, and it is desirable to avoid relaxation of the tissues which moisture would cause.

Inhalations may be indicated when there is difficulty in breathing, or when there is a dry cough, or dryness in the nose and chest. All that is required is a jug or bowl of hot water, over which the face may be held, and a towel so arranged that it covers the face below the eyes and surrounds the top of the jug. A teaspoonful of A.C.U. lotion or a pinch of salt to a pint of water should be added. This may be done for 5 to 10 minutes at bed time, or if necessary 2 or 3 times a day.

8
DIET

Diet has a twofold role in the life of man; as a means of maintaining health and as a medicine for treating the absence of health. To ensure a proper and health-giving intake of food, it is necessary to understand the basic principles of diet and to have a simple knowledge of the minerals and vitamins contained in one's daily intake.

It is generally to be observed that people do not exercise the proper control over the inputs of their bodies. We should attempt to observe our bodily habits and understand the effect, beneficial or otherwise, of the substances that constitute our daily inputs. A useful exercise is to write down everything that passes your lips for a few days. You will probably be surprised by certain eating habits which have become automatic and could be improved.

Nearly all foods which are generally available have been treated for reasons of convenience and economics, with substances which in many cases are demonstrably harmful to the body. Tinned and packaged products often contain chemical colours, preservatives, flavourings and other unnecessary substances. Most vegetables and food crops have been grown with the use of artificial fertilizers and insecticides. Animals are often treated with antibiotics, hormones and other drugs, and in the case of chickens they have often been reared under such unnatural conditions that the flavour is impaired and then restored artificially. Cases have been recorded in South America where prepubescent children were discovered to be growing breasts which were traced to the excessive female hormones passed on through the meat of their diets.

When buying foods, therefore, always remember to read the list of contents as certain additives can cause symptoms of extreme temper, hyperactivity, headaches and poor co-ordination, especially in children. In a period of a year it is possible to eat pounds in weight of chemicals which are not nutrients and simply pollute the body.

It is also surprisingly easy to manage without food that contains additives once you have made the adjustment. A list of food additives is available from the Soil Association, Walnut Tree Manor, Haughley, Stowmarket, Suffolk IP14 3RS. It is called *Look Again at the Label*, and will enable you to identify the additives and their possible effects on the system. (See also *E for Additives*, Maurice Hanssen, Thorsons, 1984.) In America a similar list is obtainable from the Food and Drug Administration.

Wash fruit and vegetables well so as to remove harmful chemical sprays. It is usually beneficial to eat the skin. What one has to avoid is the loss of substances during cooking, also the addition of such things as aluminium, lead and other substances from cooking utensils. Aluminium utensils have been proved to be harmful to health, especially when used for frying and for boiling milk and fruit. It is wise, especially when living in a city, always to make sure that children (and adults) wash their hands several times during the day and before meals to remove dust which contains lead, among other substances.

The most important factor is that one's diet should be balanced, without an excess of any single type of food. For example, meat is not essentially harmful or desirable — vegetarianism is more a matter of one's personal taste or belief — but meat, if taken, should be in moderation and preferably the non-oily variety (see Eating Guide). It also makes sense to buy, wherever possible, organically grown meat and vegetables.

Of all meats, pork has the highest ratio of fat to protein, and has also been treated against systemic parasites by the use of powerful and toxic substances; it is best avoided.

Fruit juices should not be regarded as merely a thirst quencher; they are a source of food. If you are thirsty it is better to drink water and drink juices as part of a meal. Packed juices are nowhere near as good as freshly squeezed juice, even without additives, as the packing process inevitably destroys some beneficial bacterial ingredients. Avoid drinking with meals as this dilutes the products of nutrition.

The process of preparing coffee beans is a crude form of trituration used to potentize homoeopathic remedies. The coffee grounds are, therefore, capable of counteracting any remedy that is currently being taken. If you do drink coffee at other times, never use 'instant' coffee.

High Protein Sources

Tempeh is a traditional Indonesian product. It is flat cakes made from fermented soya beans. It is now available in many countries and has not only a high quantity of protein but also a high quality protein. It has no saturated fats and is an ideal food for vegetarians as it is one of the few non-meat products that contain vitamin B_{12}. It is rich in roughage and easy to digest. Although it is fairly easy to make it does take time and needs a culture to be introduced into it and so is probably not worth making at home.

Tofu, on the other hand, is fairly easy to make at home and takes less time than making bread. Tofu is a bean curd made from the milk only of soya beans. It is also rich in high quality protein and is an excellent source of calcium and other minerals and vitamins. If you wish to try making your own tofu be sure to use beans that are less than a year old. There are excellent recipes in *Eastern Vegetarian Cooking* by Madhur Jaffrey (Cape, 1981) both for making tofu and cooking with the finished product. This book is available in the USA under the title *World of the East Vegetarian Cooking*, published by Knopf, N.Y. Another good book is *The Book of Tofu* by William Shurtleff and Akiko Aoyagi (Autumn Press, 1975).

We need proteins to burn in the fire of carbohydrates. This fire is supplemented by fats. Essentially fats are an emergency reservoir of energy that can be converted and burned as fuel. The greater the need of physical energy the more fats and carbohydrates are required. Physical work requires more fuel than mental. To reduce excess loads of body fat you need either more active physical work or to cut down on fat intake. You must also remember that carbohydrates taken in excess are stored as fat.

Fats

There are three classes of fats known as lipids which have nutritional significance as they cannot be produced within the body. The first of these are the so called fatty acids, a major source of energy in most western diets. Fatty acids may be either saturated, as they are in most meat and poultry, or unsaturated, as in most vegetable and fish oils. The degree of 'unsaturation' refers to the number of links in the molecular chain available for further chemical reactions in the body. Hence olive oil is mono-unsaturated with one such available link, whereas safflower, corn, sunflower, soy and sesame oil are polyunsaturates, containing two or more links. The essential fatty acid linoleic acid is of the polyunsaturated group, from which the body can make all the other poly-unsaturates it needs.

The second class of nutritionally significant fats includes the vitamins A, E and K, known as terpenes. Vitamin A, or Retinol, is stored in the liver and is found most notably in fish livers. It can be formed in the body from carotenes present in carrots and other plants. Vitamin K is present in greens, and is manufactured by normal bacterial flora present in the bowel. Vitamin E is present in the germs of grains and in traces in most vegetable oils. It acts as an antioxidant in these, protecting the poly-unsaturated links from breaking down (going rancid) before the plant matter has completed its life cycle. It serves the same purpose in cell membranes in our bodies, stopping the formation of 'free radicals' contributing to the formation of cancers, arterio-sclerosis and premature ageing. The term 'free radicals' denotes toxic substances which can move freely throughout the body, and have a molecular structure which enables them to bond with body tissue, possibly in places where their effect is harmful and dangerous.

The third class of nutritionally significant oils are the sterols; including cholesterol, vitamin D and incidentally the bile acids and the steroid hormones. Cholesterol is produced in the liver, bone marrow and each cell and is also present in substantial amounts in meat, milk products and eggs. It does not exist in the plant world. It cannot be utilized for energy by the body and when it is present in excess for any length of time, it can contribute to arteriosclerosis and gall stones.

Degraded poly-unsaturated fatty acids are one of the causes of scarring of the walls of small blood vessels, therefore laying the ground for future build up of cholesterol and calcium salts. This process is known as aetherio, or arteriosclerosis.

It is important to realize that polyunsaturated oils, though valuable in nutrition, can themselves become a health hazard if taken in excess or in too pure a form. They are easily degraded and can form free radicals if exposed to light, excessive heat or chemicals. Therefore they should be unrefined, cold pressed, as traces of vitamin E and other substances are present to retard such rancidity. Cold-pressed oils also contain roughage unlike processed oils. They should be stored in a cool dark place, even refrigerated. When used in cooking they should be heated slowly and never re-used. In order of preference use oils as follows:

1. Sunflower
2. Corn
3. Safflower
4. Sesame
5. Soya

Most margarines are made of unsaturated vegetable oils which are partially saturated artificially to make them solid at room temperature. This process alters them in such a way as to make them difficult for the body to use and anyway should be avoided because of the additives they always contain. Never use lard or dripping as they do not contain anything of nutritional value.

Roughage

A normal healthy diet, such as is indicated in the eating guide, will provide adequate roughage. Roughage is necessary to stimulate the colon and decreases the time that toxic substances stay in the lower intestine. Contrary to popular belief the best source of roughage is not always bran. Roughage is also found in the skins of fruit and vegetables, oatflakes, millet, barley and corn. Cabbage is not only a good source of roughage but also stimulates the beneficial bowel flora.

Those who find that their stomach is irritated by roughage can juice part of it as long as it is not strained, for example, as in soups.

These are a few basic guidelines to eating well which can be followed if in general good health but always be sure to follow any particular advice given by your physician. Never follow another patient's diet as it may not be suitable for you, and do not be persuaded into following the latest 'diet fad' of the year as it is always best to be consistent and moderate in eating. Constantly eating more than is needed can lead to health problems as can dieting when not necessary. It is sensible to rest the stomach and thus the mouth for several periods during the day so that it is not constantly working. This will aid digestion and protect the teeth (see Care of Teeth).

EATING GUIDE

1. Eat three meals a day, without haste.
2. Breakfast is the most important meal. Lunch should be medium-sized, and supper light, preferably not after 8 p.m.
3. Eat equal proportions of raw and cooked food at each meal (raw = vegetables, fruit and sprouted seed, pulses and grains). Try to eat equal quantities of chewable and non-chewable food.
4. Normally you should eat some protein with every meal, remembering that cheese and meat are not always the most favourable sources of this. For example:

Food combinations: equal proportions of any legume (lentils, peas, beans, etc.) with any grain (corn, rice, barley, oats, etc.).

Soya products: bean curd (tofu), tempeh.

Dairy products: cottage cheese, yogurt (live culture), plain hard cheeses.

Eggs: limited quantity, less than 6 per week.

Meat: poultry — non oily variety (chicken, turkey etc.); fish — with skins removed; lean lamb and beef.

(See food chart for other sources of protein.)

5. Reduce sweets: no white sugar, less brown sugar, honey, dried fruit, molasses and fruit juice.

6. Avoid excess of stimulants such as alcohol, coffee and cigarettes and never to the point of narcosis. Tobacco is harmful to the digestion as well as the rest of the body and is now well established as a cause of cancer and other diseases. Drink plenty of water, preferably between meals.

SOME USEFUL PROTEIN RECIPES

Tahini

Tahini is a paste made out of ground sesame seed. It can be made into a very smooth paste, or the seeds can be ground more lightly producing a crunchier texture. The sesame seeds should be roasted first. This can be either done in a heavy saucepan or in a special sesame seed roaster such as those used in Japan. Stir the seeds as they roast but be careful as they tend to jump out of the pan. When the sesame seeds are a shade darker take them off the heat and grind them. This can be done either in a electric grinder or with a pestle and mortar. Add in the sesame oil slowly. Use about three to one of sesame seeds to oil. Tahini can be used as a sauce with vegetables or mixed with other ingredients to make sauces or dips; for example in avocado dip or mayonnaise.

Hummus

Hummus is usually served with pitta bread but can also be spread on toast. The amount of the ingredients can be varied to suit your own taste, you may prefer more or less lemon juice or garlic.

Imperial (Metric)	American
10 oz (300g) cooked chick peas	1¼ cups cooked garbanzo beans
2 cloves garlic	2 cloves garlic
3 fl oz (100ml) lemon juice	⅓ cup lemon juice
3 tablespoons tahini	3 tablespoons tahini
Sea salt to taste	Sea salt to taste
A little water	A little water
Paprika	Paprika
Olive oil	Olive oil

1. Cook the chick peas (garbanzo beans) in a pressure cooker.

2. Put the cooked chick peas (garbanzo beans) into an electric food blender with the garlic. It is also possible to use a meat mincer or a vegetable Mouli.

3. Add the lemon juice, tahini and salt, and as much water as is needed to make the purée smooth. Blend.

4. Empty the contents into a shallow dish or deep plate and sprinkle with a little paprika. Sprinkle olive oil over the top and garnish with parsley if available.

Tisanes

The following tisanes can be used to supplement the use of China and Indian tea. All teas and tisanes should be taken weak and not too often. Never drink mint or peppermint teas as these antidote homoeopathic remedies.

Buckwheat Tea

Buckwheat is rich in rutin. You can either buy green buckwheat tea or make your own. Useful for bad circulation, cold extremities and piles. Boil the buckwheat for five minutes. This makes a pleasant tea, not unlike drinking black Indian tea.

Linden Tea

Linden tea is made from the flower of the lime tree. It is a soothing tea and so can be taken in the evening as it will not prevent sleep but may encourage it. Infuse for 5-10 minutes.

Lemon Verbena
A popular drink that has a refreshing lemon taste. Infuse for a few minutes.

Raspberry Leaf Tea
This tea has a rather grassy taste and was traditionally used to ease childbirth. It has a beneficial toning effect on the uterine muscles. Infuse for 4 minutes.

Rosehip Tea
This is a pretty red-coloured tea with a tangy taste. Rosehips have an extremely high vitamin C content; ten times as much as oranges. Infuse for 4 minutes.

Yarrow Tea
This is a lovely soothing drink which used to be very fashionable. It can be served with a slice of lemon if desired. It can be useful in gastro-intestinal conditions and for toning soft tissues. Infuse for 4 minutes.

VITAMINS

In the past an ignorance of the function of vitamins caused much suffering and death. Scurvy, beri-beri and pellagra are some of the illnesses caused by vitamin deficiencies. Until the beginning of the twentieth century it was assumed that the requirements of an adequate diet were sufficient quantities of fat, carbohydrate, protein and inorganic elements (sodium, potassium, calcium, etc.). This view changed when it was discovered that natural unrefined foods also contain organic substances that are essential to the body as catalysts in the synthesis of inorganic elements. These organic substances were called vitamins.

In 1969, the *International Journal of Vitamin Research* offered the following definition: 'A vitamin is an organic substance of a nutritive nature which is present in low concentrations as a natural compound of enzyme systems, and catalyzes required reactions, and may be derived externally to the tissues or intrinsic biosynthesis.'

Many vitamins act as co-enzymes or as a prosthetic, supporting groups of enzymes responsible for promoting essential chemical reactions. They regulate the metabolism, helping to convert fat and carbohydrate into energy, and assist in forming bones and tissues. Some are relatively simple, while others are quite complex. Fats, proteins and elements can be changed and converted in the body; stored fat which can be converted into carbohydrate, and carbohydrate which can be converted and stored as fat, are examples. However, with only a few exceptions, the body is unable to synthesize vitamins. Therefore they must be supplied regularly in the diet.

Vitamins can be classified as either water-soluble or fat-soluble. Water-soluble vitamins may be dissolved in the cooking water and are destroyed by over-cooking. They are not normally stored in the body; that which is not required is excreted in the urine. Therefore we require a regular daily supply of water-soluble vitamins. Fat-soluble vitamins are fairly stable in cooking. They are not lost in the cooking water when heated and are not excreted in the urine. Antibiotics, mineral oils such as liquid paraffin, and various other drugs interfere with their absorption from the intestinal tract. In cases of excess fat-soluble vitamins, water-soluble vitamins are retained by the body to counteract the ill-effects of the former. A vitamin abundance can become an excess of vitamins in a diet; too much may have just as undesirable consequences as too little.

Supplementation?

The most recent research shows no justification for indiscriminate use of vitamin tablets — a fashion so grown out of all proportions to reality. At best a thorough knowledge of the function of vitamins is necessary and small doses can sometimes be taken for a limited time when minor deficiencies are suspected. The inter-relationship of vitamins within the metabolic system is a highly complex situation. If you increase C beyond a certain point, A and D are used up. Increase E beyond a certain point and you immediately reduce B_{12}. Too much B_1 reduces the action of C and E. Everything is inter-related. There are no separate bits which can be manipulated for expedient advantage.

Vitamins are in essence catalysts which ensure the proper action of enzymes. Within a metabolic situation where an ordinary diet is being properly absorbed, the enzymes feed the body. The situation is one of symbiosis and the vitamins are only the catalysts facilitating the operation of the two partners to the symbiosis: the body supporting the enzymes and the enzymes supporting the body.

If you overdose with catalysts at any point you will either overproduce co-enzymes or break up enzymes. The balance is most delicate and the oversupply of vitamins means a break-down in the system — because the enzymes are subjected to catalytic action beyond their tolerance to support.

In 1970, Yudkin showed that vitamin deficiency can exist in a situation of vitamin abundance. He conducted a clinical study and research into vitamin B deficiencies in children. The following was the result of a mixture of all vitamin B constituents being given to some of the sick children and a similar tablet with nothing in it to others:

	Observer	No Change	Better	Worse
Tablet	B	12	2	0
	Y	11	2	0
Placebo	B	12	4	3
	Y	14	3	2

The results show no significant change. The simple truth is that vitamin deficiency has an anterior causation in the absorption mechanism. If the absorption mechanism fails, oral administration of vitamins leads to no change. It is absorption that should be studied and improved.

In brief, vitamin supplements can be highly dangerous and should be administered only within the limits of a fragile metabolic balance which only a doctor can hope to assess. When gross deficiency is suspected in acute or chronic illness it is the function of biological study, with the aid perhaps of a pathologist, to establish why absorption failed, in what form vitamins are to be used and with what dosage. The woman behind the counter of the health food shop, however well-intentioned, is *not* qualified to do this.

Another major problem is the fortifying of foods with vitamins. Before and during the second world war cod liver oil was added to the diet of school children. Then an investigation by the British Paediatric Association showed that fewer people were using National cod liver oil than had been expected. As a result, better prophylactic measures were advised and National dried milk for babies was introduced, fortified 280 I.U. per ounce. Cod liver oil was also fortified to 200 I.U. (5 mg) per gram.

All was thought to be well until Lightwood in 1952 diagnosed hypercalcaemia. Babies and children became obviously ill; they had high blood calcium and deposits of metabolic calcium, especially in the kidneys and also at times in the lungs, brain, blood vessels, etc. At this time mothers were receiving vitamins A and D, and babies their fortified milk and cereals, and cod liver oil. Add to this the natural synthesis of vitamin D by sunlight and one has a dangerous situation on hand. It was then advised that all the above should be reduced. However, even now hypercalcaemia has not been totally eliminated, although it is very rare.

In some countries bananas are fortified with vitamin D, oranges with vitamin D and flour with vitamin B_1. We force ripen various fruits by picking them before they have ripened naturally. As they have less 'nutrition value' than if they ripened naturally, vitamins are then added without creating or considering the natural balance. We whiten the flour of natural wheat extraction, thereby removing all native vitamin B and some native minerals. An enrichment is added because we cannot be bothered educating people not to eat white flour. In 1942, 38% of British millers added thiamine (synthetic) to white flour. War necessitated maximum use of home-made wheat, and extraction beyond 85% was forbidden with the result that the need to add thiamin disappeared. But when war was over we went back to 1942 habits.

Although we add major lost vitamins, we still do not make up the minor vitamin and mineral losses. Nor do we educate people to eat better.

Potatoes are an important source of vitamin C. We now sell and feed people on sophisticated potatoes which have been peeled, left to soak, dried, heated, mashed — murdered — without any consideration. A hospital survey in 1963 stated: 'potatoes as served in most hospitals do not make any substantial contribution to the provision of ascorbic acid'.

A similar situation is found with orange juices, citrus juices and soft drinks with cyclamates. All these wean people away from oranges, apples, lemons, honeys and natural sources of nourishment and vitamins.

Good news is the increasing use of proteins from soya beans, leaf protein and algae.

Vegans, those who do not eat or use any product derived from an animal source, are becoming conscious of the lack of vitamin B_{12} which is found mainly in animal food. A good source of non-animal vitamin B_{12} is in tempeh flatcake made of fermented soya beans.

Good nutrition relies on a proper understanding of the body's need for vitamins and the means by which they are supplied and absorbed into the system.

Study the description given below of the various vitamins and their effect on the body. Try to identify any symptoms of deficiencies which will prevent the absorption of energies. The city dweller will be especially prone to vitamin deficiencies. Locate the vitamin you think it may be necessary to take and then discuss this and any deficiencies with your doctor.

Vitamin A (Retinol) Fat-soluble
Vitamin A is a pale yellow crystalline substance chemically defined as an alcohol. As the name retinol suggests it has a vital function relating to the retina of the eye. Its presence is essential for seeing in the dark and for seeing colours.

Vitamin A plays a vital role in protein utilization and is therefore essential for tooth formation, and for the growth of bone and soft tissues. The formation and maintenance of mucous membranes, which help the body's natural defences against infection, are dependent on vitamin A, as are normal reproduction and lactation.

Being fat-soluble it is stored in the body. The main sites are the lungs, kidneys and the liver. The liver, which stores about 90% of the total amount necessary for a normal state of health, accumulates a reserve which is built up during the growth years.

Sources. Natural sources of vitamin A are liver, kidneys, egg yolk, dark green leaves, and dairy products such as butter. Therapeutic doses can be obtained from cod and halibut liver oils. Red fruits and root vegetables, especially carrots, contain alpha and gamma carotenes, which are converted by co-enzymes in the intestinal tract into provitamin A. This provitamin is then converted by the liver into vitamin A.

Deficiency and toxicity effects. An intake of much below 20 I.U. (6 mg) per kg body weight of vitamin A per day will cause deficiency symptoms. Vitamin A deficiency, particularly in children and in pregnancy, is one of the most common nutritional diseases. Its main effect is night-blindness, which can develop into the more serious xerophthalinia, a severe inflammation.

Normal diets usually contain adequate quantities of vitamin A; however, childhood and pregnancy require more of the foods which contain high levels of the vitamin. Toxicity does not occur from food intakes unless one takes massive doses from polar bear liver oils or large quantities of cod liver oils. Overdoses in excess of 50,000 I.U. daily produce the effects of growth stunting, bone fragility, pain, eczema and enlargement of the liver and spleen.

Stability. As it is fat-soluble, the vitamin is fairly stable in cooking; with meat and fish one should be careful not to cook away too much of the juice leaving behind only dry, fibrous tissues. Some vitamin A is lost in sun drying, oxidation and freezing processes.

Signs of deficiency or excess of intake. Poor reactions while driving at night; softening of the cornea; dry, scaly or rough skin, known as 'goose' or 'toad' skin, may point to a vitamin A deficiency, but also possibly to a B-complex deficiency.

In the laboratory, photometric tests to determine one's adaptations and reactions in the dark are used to detect vitamin A deficiencies. Response to dosage is fast, a return to equilibrium can be achieved usually after only a few days' treatment.

B-Complex Vitamins

There are many vitamins in the B-complex group. They are treated as a group because there is such an interdependence between the action of all the individual compounds that they must be supplied together and in their proper proportions. The therapeutic use of only a single member of the group can cause deficiency in another of the group. Vitamins A, D and E act in much the same way. Powdered yeast has the most suitable proportions of the group and is therefore the best source of vitamin B-complex.

Vitamin B₁ (Thiamin) Water-soluble

The pure vitamin is a yellowish crystalline powder with a salty taste. It is essential for tissue respiration and the metabolism of fats, proteins and carbohydrates. As it is water-soluble and therefore not stored in the body in any appreciable quantities, vitamin B_1 must be supplied to the system daily. Excess is excreted in the urine.

Sources. Some of the vitamin is synthesized in the intestines, although the amount available from this source is small. Animals produce higher quantities.

Wheat germ, yeast powder, beans, peas, whole grains, fresh lean pork and all organ meats such as liver, heart etc., are good sources of B-complex. Dairy products, fruit and vegetables contain very little B-complex.

Deficiency and toxicity effects. Severe deficiency can affect the nervous system and reflex responses. Progressive deterioration can end in paralysis and atrophy of involuntary muscles. Thus, it can cause degeneration of the heart muscles and cardiac failure. Also atrophy of the intestinal tract leading to decreased hydrochloric acid secretion in the stomach causing anorexia (loss of appetite). In the large intestine it could cause stasis leading to constipation. These are all typical symptoms of beri-beri.

Constant exercise, fever and hyperthyroid activity are conditions requiring a greater intake of B_1. Older people require a greater intake of the vitamin B group because they utilize it less efficiently. There are no known toxic effects. Vitamin B deficiencies are quite common in the West.

Stability. Considerable losses of vitamin B occur in cooking. This is dependent upon the amount of water used and discarded, if any additives have been used to preserve the food for long periods of time, and upon the acidity of the food. The higher the acidity of the food, as in the addition of vinegar, lemons etc. while cooking, the lower the vitamin B content.

Vitamin B_2 (Riboflavin) Water-soluble
Riboflavin is a solid, crystalline, yellow, fluorescent substance. It is a catalyst for glucose and fat assimilation, and therefore essential to growth. It is absorbed into the system through the small intestine but it is not stored in the body.

Sources. Most foods contain B_2. The best sources are milk, cottage and cheddar cheese, lean meats and green leafy vegetables.

Deficiency and toxicity effects. Ariboflavinosis is the disease caused by vitamin B_2 deficiency. Symptoms are cracks in the skin at the corner of the mouth, a purplish tongue and growths in the corner of the eyes.

Stability. Riboflavin is easily lost by exposure to light, especially ultra-violet light. However, due partly to its low solubility in water, it is stable to heat, oxidation and acid.

Vitamin B_6 (Pyridoxine) Water-soluble
B_6 is a complex in itself of three different compounds that are called pyridoxine. It is a white crystalline inter-related compound which is soluble in water or alcohol. It is absorbed in the upper small intestine. It plays an essential role in the body's food metabolizing processes. It functions as a co-enzyme so as to metabolize protein.

It also plays a part in the release of glycogerol, an aspect of sugar, from the liver and muscles.

Sources. The richest sources are wheat germ, yeast, pork and glandular meats, especially liver, whole grains, legumes and potatoes.

Deficiency and toxicity effects. As with the other B vitamins, deficiency effects arise from insufficient intakes in one's daily diet. Laboratory tests have shown that certain drugs, such as izioniazid, which is used for tubercular patients, are antagonists which deactivate the vitamin.

Vitamin C (Ascorbic Acid) Water-soluble

Vitamin C is a hexose derivative and is classified as a carbohydrate. The main function of carbohydrates is to provide essential heat to the body. This heat protects the body from infection and helps it to repair its injuries. Therefore, repair of the body requires heat and lack of infection. Growth of the body also requires heat.

It is the function of vitamin C as a chemical to help in better utilization of carbohydrates. It is therefore a growth-providing and anti-infective vitamin. It is necessary for the healing of all broken tissues, broken bones, cuts, sores, bruises etc. It prevents the blood from escaping from small vessels, both superficial and deep, by acting as a catalyst in calcium and vitamin D absorption. Vitamin C also promotes absorption of any vitamin B which has been derived from vegetable sources.

Vitamin C is absorbed from the small intestines and is carried to the tissues by the blood. It is stored in the adrenal glands, the liver, spleen and the kidneys. A daily supply is necessary to maintain its preventative effects. Excess amounts are excreted in the urine and in the faeces.

Sources. Vitamin C is found in citrus fruits, tomatoes and leafy vegetables. Although they contain less of the vitamin, potatoes form an important source when a regular part of the diet. Dairy products and meat contain almost no vitamin C.

Deficiency and toxicity effects. The primary deficiency effect of vitamin C is scurvy. This was prevalent among sailors and soldiers until oranges or limes were found to prevent it. General debility, poor appetite, sensitivity to touch, joint pains and swollen and bleeding gums are all symptoms of the disease. Other deficiency symptoms are discolouring of areas of the skin through haemorrhaging of small blood vessels and, in some cases, stools may become bloody.

Since the introduction of the potato into our diet, the occurence of vitamin C deficiency is rare. However, unless care is taken certain specialist diets undertaken without the guidance of a physician can result in a vitamin C deficiency. Also, babies who are constantly fed by artificial means are susceptible to it.

Large doses (1g) can be beneficial in curing colds and fighting infection. These can be obtained in warm lemon and honey drinks or citrus fruits. Extra vitamin C is certainly needed in illness, especially fever, to maintain tissue levels. Cigarette smokers need twice as much of the vitamin to maintain the same level in the tissues as a non smoker. The reason for this is quite complicated but the chemistry of it has been traced.

Excessive doses are harmful to the kidneys, to the vitamin A and calcium metabolism, and have been shown to be the possible cause of urate, cystine or oxalate stones in the kidneys and gall bladder.

In cases of acute illness, I advocate a large dose (1g) followed every few hours by a small maintenance dose (100mg).

Stability. Vitamin C is the most easily lost of all vitamins. As it is water-soluble, it is dissolved in cooking water and is oxidized by heat and air, especially in the presence of copper or an alkaline solution. Bruising, cutting, freezing, storing and sodium bicarbonate used in cooking all cause loss of vitamin C.

Deficiency symptoms. Tendency to bruise easily, wounds infecting easily and taking a long time to heal, bloody diarrhoea and blotchy areas of the skin, poor appetite and sensitivity to touch, are all signs of a deficiency.

In the laboratory, analysis of the levels of vitamin C in the plasma are used as a means of determining vitamin C deficiency. Levels of below 0.2mg per 100mg are scurvy-causing.

Vitamin D — Fat-soluble

As vitamin D is synthesized by the body with the aid of sunlight, it cannot be accurately defined as a vitamin. However, vitamin D regulates and maintains the levels of calcium and phosphorus in the body and the rate at which these minerals are absorbed and secreted in the bones. It is therefore essential for normal growth and important for bone and tooth formation.

As with vitamin A, vitamin D is stored in the fatty deposits of the body, as well as in the liver, skin, bones and brain.

Sources. Most of the vitamin D we utilize comes from the action of sunlight on a provitamin contained in the skin, thereby forming vitamin D_2. In foods, the richest source of vitamin D_3 is fish oils. It is also found in vegetable and animal oils, and small quantities in dairy products.

Deficiency and toxicity effects. The most recognizable effect of vitamin D deficiency is rickets, which is found particularly in children. Lack of the vitamin affects absorption of calcium in the intestine and therefore results in failure of the bones to appropriate or retain calcium. This results in softened, weakened bones, showing as bending and enlargement deformities.

Osteomalacia (bone deformities) is an associated illness that is sometimes caused by a vitamin D deficiency. Its symptoms are similar to those of rickets: bone weaknesses and deformities, especially in the limbs and spine; physical weakness and rheumatic type pains, two symptoms found particularly in pregnant women.

Prevention and cure of rickets and osteomalacia requires adequate provision of calcium and phosphorus (see food values chart), as well as vitamin D_2. Usually, deficiency only occurs if the person is habitually shielded from sunlight. However, excessive taking of baths can also result in insufficient vitamin D formation due to lack of provitamin D on the skin. This can be remedied by doses of fish liver oils.

Weakness, headache, nausea, vomiting and diarrhoea, kidney-stones and high blood-pressure are all symptoms of toxicity which can occur in babies and children who have been given excessive doses of vitamin pills and liveroils.

Stability. Vitamin D is very stable, both in cooking and in processing.

Signs of deficiency or excess in intake. Deficiency signs are: profuse sweating and restlessness, bowing of the legs in infants, and, in elderly people, rheumatic pain and general weakness.

Evidence of deficiency is shown in laboratory tests by an increase of calcium in the urine followed by an increase of calcium in the stools. The quantity of phosphorus excreted may also be increased at the same time.

Vitamin E — Fat-soluble

This vitamin was originally associated with the process of reproduction and was therefore named tocopherol from the Greek word meaning offspring.

In the system, vitamin E helps create a balance between vitamins A and C and also maintains and protects that balance by preventing their destruction or excretion by the digestive processes. It also serves a balancing function, controlling the proportions of vitamins A, C and E within the system. There is evidence to suggest that vitamin E can help lungs damaged by smoke and give some protection against air pollution.

The role that vitamin E plays in the ageing process and sexual functions has probably been exaggerated by commercial marketers of vitamin supplements. Excessive extrapolation from results noted in experiments on animals is often taken as justification for their claims.

Unlike the other fat-soluble vitamins, vitamin E is not stored in the liver but in other fatty deposits of the body, such as the kidneys or the buttocks. The pituitary and adrenal glands also have a high concentration of the vitamin.

Sources. High concentrations are found in wheat germ oil and other cereal germs. Green plants, dairy products, liver and vegetable oils contain vitamin E, and chemists have now managed to produce it by a chemical process.

Deficiency and toxicity effects. Severe vitamin E deficiencies are seldom found, as adequate amounts of it are generally present in the human diet and it can also be stored for long periods in body tissues.

Although experiments on animals have produced many deficiency symptoms, no conclusive parallels can be drawn. Toxic effects from large quantities are very rare, but high potency supplements can cause headaches, nausea and giddiness. Patients with high blood-pressure should always start taking vitamin E at a low dosage and increase slowly.

Stability. It is quite stable in cooking except when in contact with lead or iron. Rancid fat destroys vitamin E, as does deep-freezing. Any rancidity of the oil used as a source (e.g. wheat germ oil) means that the vitamin E is lost.

Vitamin K — Fat-soluble

All the forms of vitamin K belong to the group known as quinones. There are two types of quinones: K and K_2. The first is found in green plants, and the second is a natural product of bacterial action in the intestinal tract. Vitamin K plays a highly complex and essential role which is not yet fully understood.

Vitamin K was originally known as the 'coagulatory' vitamin due to the discovery that its properties are connected with the prevention of haemorrhaging. It synthesizes various proteins in the liver which are essential for the proper clotting of blood. Vitamin K prevents the formation of adhesions and scars in wounds. The body does not store the vitamin in any appreciable quantity.

Sources. Sufficient quantities of vitamin K are found in the average diets of adults and children to preclude any deficiencies. Should one occur due to a very inadequate diet, poor coagulation of the blood and persistent bruising will result. Sometimes, if a nursing mother has been having anti-coagulant therapy, the baby may need a small (1mg) dose to prevent bruising.

Food sources of vitamin K are cabbage, spinach, lettuce, wheat germ, tomatoes, oil, eggs, and liver.

In the USA it is not sold over the counter as large doses can cause toxicity.

Stability. There is usually little loss in cooking, but sunlight can destroy vitamin K.

MINERALS

Trace elements needed in the body in minute or fairly small quantities

Cobalt	Molybdenum
Copper	Nickel
Fluorine	Selenium
Manganese	Vanadium

Calcium

Calcium is the most abundant mineral in the body found mainly in the bones and teeth. It is necessary for the structures of bones and teeth and has a catalytic function in muscular growth and activity and nerve transmission. Calcium absorption is very inefficient and is affected by a wide range of factors; the presence of vitamins A,

C and D are essential to absorption. Lack of exercise and stress also affect absorption. The action of calcium in the body is wide ranging and therefore not possible to list here in full detail.

Sources. Tofu, milk, yogurt, cheese and fish (including the backbone).

Deficiency and toxicity effects. When the body finds itself short of calcium, because it is losing more via the kidneys than it is gaining from the food, it draws on its store in the bones and teeth. There is often a deficiency during pregnancy and old age. Deficiency can result in bone and teeth disturbances, cramps, joint pains, insomnia and irritability of nerves and muscles. High intake of calcium and vitamin D may result in excessive calcification of the bones and tissues.

Chlorine
Chlorine is widely distributed throughout the body and helps to regulate the correct balance of acid and alkali in the blood. It also stimulates the liver to function as a filter for wastes and toxins and therefore keep the system clean.

Sources. Chlorine is provided almost exclusively in salt but is also found in kelp, rye flour, ripe olives and sea greens.

Deficiency and toxicity effects. It is extremely rare for a deficiency to occur as salt is found so widely in the normal diet. An excess of chlorine can destroy vitamin E and many of the beneficial bowel flora.

Iodine
Most of iodine is converted into iodide in the body and stored in the thyroid gland. Iodide plays an important role in regulating the body's production of energy, promoting growth and stimulating the rate of metabolism. The thyroid gland influences the condition of hair, nails, skin, teeth and affects speech and mentality. It also inhibits the conversion of carotene to vitamin A if not functioning properly.

Sources. Sea fish, sea weeds, watercress.

Deficiency and toxicity effects. Deficiency results in thyroid enlargement and hypothyroidism. It may also lead to hardening of the arteries, obesity, slow metabolism, palpitations, nervousness and irritability. If a mother is deficient in iodine during adolescence and pregnancy her child could be born with physical and mental retardation, which can be helped if treated immediately. Toxicity does not usually occur unless iodine is overprescribed as a medicine, where it can be serious.

Iron
Iron is a necessary part of the red pigment in blood called haemoglobin. Haemoglobin transports oxygen in the blood to the tissues to maintain healthy life functions. Iron is also necessary for muscle contraction and is stored mainly in the liver, spleen, bone marrow and blood. The balance of calcium, phosphorus and iron is very important. Women have a greater need of iron because of loss in menstruation, and particularly in pregnancy.

Sources. Much of iron found in food cannot be utilized by the body, for example, in spinach. Good sources of iron include leafy green vegetables, lean meat, tongue, liver and black treacle.

Deficiency and toxicity effects. It is difficult to know how much iron is 'enough' as the body can keep a reserve in the spleen and liver for use in deficiency. Evidence indicates that 'naturally' occurring ferrous iron is used more efficiently in the body. It would seem that it is better to increase intake of foods rich in iron than to take iron supplements which tend to be indigestible. Vitamin E aids the assimilation of iron and vitamin C will speed up the restoration of haemoglobin levels to normal.

Magnesium
70 per cent of magnesium is found in the bones and 30 per cent is found in the soft tissues and body fluids. Magnesium is involved in many essential metabolic processes. It helps promote absorption and metabolism of minerals such as calcium, phosphorus, sodium, B complex vitamins and vitamins C and E. Magnesium is needed in the conversion of blood sugar into energy.

Sources. Nearly every food contains some magnesium but rich sources are fresh green vegetables, soya beans, figs, corn and apples.

Deficiency and toxicity effects. Deficiency can occur in the case of diabetics and alcoholics or in any case of severe malabsorption. Symptoms caused by deficiency may include muscle twitching, confusion, disorientation and the formation of clots in the heart and brain. Large amounts of magnesium can be toxic especially if the calcium intake is low and the phosphorus intake high.

Phosphorus
Phosphorus is the second most abundant mineral in the body and because it is present in every cell, plays a part in almost every chemical reaction within the body. It is necessary for proper growth of bones and teeth, kidney functioning and nerve transmission.

Sources. The role of phosphorus is closely related to that of calcium. As long as enough calcium is taken in the diet phosphorus will not be lacking. Phosphorus is found in all foods that contain calcium (although not the other way round) and is easily absorbed. Other sources are meat, fish, eggs and whole grains.

Deficiency and toxicity effects. A deficiency in phosphorus is rare unless the calcium/phosphorus/vitamin D balance is disturbed, but it could lead to weight changes, irregular breathing, fatigue and mental disorders. There is no known toxicity of phosphorus.

Potassium
Potassium is found mainly in the intercellular fluid where it helps regulate the distribution of fluids on both sides of the cell walls. It also helps in the conversion of glucose to glycogen for storage in the liver. It is necessary for normal growth, cell metabolism and to stimulate the kidneys to eliminate toxic body wastes. The action of potassium and sodium are closely linked.

Sources. Potatoes (especially the skins), bananas, green leafy vegetables, oranges and whole grains.

Deficiency and toxicity effects. Deficiency mainly occurs when there is high body fluid loss, e.g. from vomiting, diarrhoea, excess urination or sweating. Potassium absorption is affected by white sugar, alcohol, coffee and hormone drugs such as cortisone. Symptoms of deficiency include weakness, poor reflexes, sagging muscles and acne in youth and dry skin in older persons. There is no known toxicity of potassium.

Sodium
Fifty per cent of sodium is found in extracellular fluids and the rest in the bones. Many of its functions are carried out in conjunction with phosphorus. An important function of sodium is to keep the

blood minerals soluble so they do not form deposits in the bloodstream.

Sources. Sodium is found in virtually all foods but especially salt, seafoods, carrots and kelp.

Deficiency and toxicity effects. Deficiency is rare as the usual intake of sodium is far higher than necessary, but it can occur if physical work is consistently carried out in high temperatures. In this case muscle shrinkage, weight loss, rheumatism and neuralgia may occur. An excess of sodium is much more common and causes abnormal fluid retention, high blood-pressure and dizziness.

Sulphur
Sulphur is a non-metallic element that is found in every cell of animals and plants. It helps oxygen and other substances to build cells and release energy. It is closely linked with protein and keeps skin, nails and hair healthy.

Sources. Sulphur is found in foods containing protein, such as meat, fish, legumes and nuts, but also in cabbage, Brussels sprouts and dried beans.

Deficiency and toxicity effects. If enough protein is ingested the level of sulphur will be adequate. Intake of 'non organic' sulphur may lead to toxicity.

Zinc
Zinc is stored in many parts of the body but is found in the largest quantities in the liver, pancreas, kidneys, bones and voluntary muscles. It has many functions and is essential for growth and the proper development of the reproductive organs and the prostate gland. Zinc influences the absorption of B complex vitamins and is involved with many enzymes to do with digestion and metabolism.

Sources. Most foods but especially whole grain products, yeast and pumpkin seeds.

Deficiency and toxicity effects. Deficiency may cause stunted growth, sexual immaturity, slow wound healing and poor appetite with loss of taste. Toxicity does not normally occur except where food has been stored in galvanized containers.

FOOD CONTENTS VALUES

The charts given below show the vitamin and protein values of the foods we commonly eat. You can work out what proportion of your daily intake is provided in each category.

Category 1. Raw juicy fruits. Perfect synthesis of fire, air and water. Ideal food for the intellectual and sedentary worker, more so in warm seasons and warm climates.

Category 2. Complementary to category 1; deals with liquid content of human body.

Category 3. Not of eliminative, but of building foods. The organic contents that contribute to the building of bones — the rest are muscle builders. They are excellent food for manual functions and in cold seasons and climates.

Category 4. Dried, sweet and oily fruits, milk products and eggs are concentrated products. They are heat-producing and, above all, nourishing foods. In excess they are fattening, more so to the intellectual and sedentary person.

Category 5. Useless as foods, but good as bulk builders, and useful for nervous people with manageable appetites. Note that dry legumes and pulses should be well cooked to get their protein, or should be sprouted.

COMPOSITION OF MINERAL MATTER IN 1,000 PARTS OF WATER FREE SUBSTANCE

CONSTITUTION OF THE HUMAN BODY AND ITS PARTS

Names of Parts of Body and of Foods	Predominant Radiations	Predominant Vitamins	Calories per 100 Grams	Water	Protein	Fat	Carbohydrates (Sugar, Starch)	Mineral Matter	Potassium K_2O	Sodium Na_2O	Calcium CaO	Magnesium MgO	Iron Fe_2O_3	Phosphorus P_2O_5	Sulphur SO_3	Silicon SiO_2	Chlorine	Fluorine	Total
HUMAN BODY, WHOLE	HR	ABCDE	—	60.00	19.00	15.00	1.00	5.00	3.30	3.00	70.50	2.15	0.70	32.15	4.10	1.00	7.00	1.10	125.00
RED BLOOD CORPUSCLES	〃	〃	—	68.78	30.20	—	—	1.02	13.81	5.87	0.55	0.30	5.00	3.50	0.28	0.01	5.68	—	35.00
BLOOD PLASMA	〃	〃	—	90.00	9.00	—	0.15	0.85	3.30	36.75	3.20	2.35	—	1.75	1.45	0.22	36.20	—	85.22
BLOOD SERUM	〃	〃	—	90.75	8.24	—	0.15	0.86	3.60	41.80	3.50	2.45	—	1.60	1.55	0.50	40.00	—	94.72
LYMPH	〃	〃	—	94.82	4.00	0.40	0.05	0.73	3.93	57.88	1.17	0.31	0.06	1.32	—	0.36	54.75	—	119.92
LUNGS	〃	〃	—	79.25	15.20	3.65	—	1.90	1.24	24.70	1.80	3.04	0.36	46.07	1.32	0.07	6.17	—	85.00
BRAIN	〃	〃	—	81.10	8.50	9.30	—	1.10	19.50	6.80	0.40	0.70	0.16	27.30	0.42	0.14	4.35	—	59.70
LIVER	〃	〃	—	71.55	20.00	3.65	3.25	1.55	13.90	7.90	1.97	0.11	1.44	27.30	0.50	0.11	1.26	—	54.52
SPLEEN	〃	〃	—	76.14	17.10	4.20	1.00	1.56	6.12	28.26	4.77	0.30	4.64	17.26	1.55	0.21	0.35	—	63.36
BILE	〃	〃	—	89.00				0.85	2.88	30.35	0.85	0.32	—	6.27	3.83	—	15.06	—	59.91
BONES, FRESH	〃	〃	—	Water and fat-free substance					—	—	240.00	8.00	10.00	345.00	—	—	12.00	15.00	630.00
MUSCLE TISSUE, FRESH	〃	〃	—	75.50	18.70	3.70	1.00	1.10	18.00	2.80	0.40	1.80	0.20	22.00	0.60	0.40	2.80	—	49.00
HUMAN MILK	〃	〃	66	87.75	1.60	3.95	6.25	0.45	11.73	3.16	5.80	0.75	0.07	7.84	0.33	0.07	6.38	—	36.13

CATEGORY 1

GROUP A — 50% OF THE DAILY RATION — RAW JUICE FRUITS — STRONGLY ELIMINATIVE FOODS

Names of Parts of Body and of Foods	Predominant Radiations	Predominant Vitamins	Calories per 100 Grams	Water	Protein	Fat	Carbohydrates (Sugar, Starch)	Mineral Matter	Potassium K_2O	Sodium Na_2O	Calcium CaO	Magnesium MgO	Iron Fe_2O_3	Phosphorus P_2O_5	Sulphur SO_3	Silicon SiO_2	Chlorine	Fluorine	Total
APPLE	CR	BE	61	85.60	0.40	0.50	13.00	0.50	11.78	8.61	1.35	2.89	0.46	4.52	2.01	1.42	—	—	33.04
PEAR	〃	〃	63	84.40	0.60	0.10	14.10	0.40	14.00	2.17	2.05	1.52	0.25	3.90	1.45	0.38	—	—	25.72
PEACH	〃	〃	65	89.32	0.70	—	9.40	0.48	20.90	3.00	4.60	1.35	0.50	6.05	3.50	2.80	0.80	—	40.70
APRICOT	〃	〃	61	84.70	1.42	—	13.34	0.54	19.68	3.76	1.08	1.22	0.26	3.76	0.92	0.68	0.20	—	33.58
PLUM	〃	〃	76	78.40	1.00	—	20.00	0.60	16.45	0.15	2.78	1.53	0.90	4.17	1.03	1.19	—	—	27.69
PRUNE, FRESH	〃	〃	40	82.00	0.80	—	16.50	0.70	18.28	3.41	4.34	1.36	0.94	6.03	1.21	—	0.15	—	36.91
NECTARINE	〃	〃	39	82.90	0.60	—	15.90	0.60	—	—	—	—	—	—	—	—	—	—	—

ABBREVIATIONS: C = Cosmic   S = Solar   T = Terrestrial   H = Human   A = Animal   R = Radiations

Food	Code	BE	No.	%	(1)	(2)	(3)	(4)	(5)	(6)	(7)	(8)	(9)	(10)	(11)	(12)	(13)	(14)	Total
GROUP B																			
STRAWBERRY	SR		44	89.90	1.00	0.60	7.70	0.80	13.72	18.53	9.23	—	3.73	7.97	2.05	7.83	1.10	—	64.16
RASPBERRY, BLACK	::		62	84.10	1.70	1.00	12.60	0.60	16.50	1.90	3.15	1.75	0.05	4.50	11.50	—	—	—	42.35
RASPBERRY, RED	::		62	88.70	1.00	—	16.60	0.60	26.44	3.00	3.70	2.82	0.50	8.05	1.44	—	2.90	—	46.37
HUCKLEBERRY	::		55	81.00	0.80	0.60	11.30	1.00	12.10	0.04	1.46	0.95	0.03	2.17	7.95	0.42	—	—	25.05
CURRANT, RED	:CR		61	87.95	0.30	—	13.60	0.45	16.90	0.16	0.29	0.45	0.05	1.40	3.95	—	0.35	—	23.50
CURRANT, WHITE	::		61	85.56	0.40	—	18.70	0.44	13.70	0.13	0.60	0.75	0.04	2.27	0.90	—	0.30	—	22.30
CURRANT, BLACK	::		61	79.79	1.00	1.00	10.90	0.51	17.90	0.60	7.95	4.75	0.05	6.20	1.71	—	0.08	—	40.15
BLACKBERRY	:SR		42	86.35	1.30	—	8.40	0.45	11.22	2.87	3.54	0.90	1.32	3.54	14.20	0.75	1.80	—	29.04
GOOSEBERRY	CR		55	90.70	0.50	0.60	8.40	0.40	9.00	0.03	10.15	—	0.04	1.60	—	—	0.22	—	35.95
CRANBERRY	CR			90.20	0.40	—	—	0.40	—	—	—	—	—	—	—	—	0.03	—	—
MULBERRY	CR		38	84.70	0.50	0.30	14.30	0.60	13.50	1.80	1.40	1.20	0.35	4.80	1.05	—	0.15	—	24.25
MEDLAR	::		103	82.10	0.60	—	16.50	0.46	74.50	6.45	12.55	—	1.84	18.41	2.34	—	6.81	—	126.36
MIRABELLE	::		32	85.34	0.60	0.70	13.60	0.70	18.75	0.40	2.70	1.25	0.45	4.00	1.50	3.46	0.35	—	30.00
RHUBARB (JUICE)	:SR		18	94.40	0.60	1.25	3.60	0.65	17.94	0.76	2.60	1.90	0.70	5.54	1.76	0.60	0.48	—	34.59
GRAPE	CR		40	78.20	1.30	0.80	18.60	0.70	8.00	12.25	1.65	0.90	0.06	2.50	0.20	3.11	0.34	—	25.90
CHERRY	::		77	80.80	1.00	1.60	16.70	0.70	—	—	—	—	—	—	—	—	—	—	—
POMEGRANATE	::		7	79.50	1.50	1.60	16.80	0.60	—	—	—	—	—	—	—	—	—	—	—
FIG, FRESH (BLACK)	:SR		81	79.50	1.50	0.20	18.70	0.60	18.00	3.75	4.00	2.10	1.75	5.60	2.10	1.60	1.10	—	40.00
WATERMELON	::		32	92.30	0.50	0.20	6.70	0.30	—	—	—	—	—	—	—	—	—	—	—
MUSKMELON	::		30	91.60	0.60	—	7.20	0.60	—	—	—	—	—	—	—	—	—	—	—
GROUP C																			
LEMON	CR		44	89.30	1.00	0.70	8.50	0.50	22.54	0.84	12.75	2.09	0.20	5.25	1.25	0.31	0.18	—	45.41
LIME	::		44	97.61	0.83	—	0.58	0.98	28.38	—	5.17	1.56	—	5.70	2.24	—	2.65	—	45.70
ORANGE	::		51	86.90	0.80	0.20	11.60	0.39	18.62	0.95	8.65	2.03	0.38	4.70	2.00	0.25	0.29	—	37.87
GRAPEFRUIT	::		48	91.68	0.56	—	7.37	0.56	13.20	—	2.20	1.20	0.38	3.32	1.00	—	0.40	—	21.70
MANGO	::		80	88.60	0.60	0.40	9.90	—	18.95	—	2.55	0.64	—	2.60	1.47	—	1.55	—	27.76
PAPAYA	::		4	88.59	0.50	0.05	29.70	—	—	—	—	—	—	—	—	—	—	—	—
PERSIMMON	::			67.90	0.80	0.30	9.70	—	—	—	—	—	—	—	—	—	—	—	—
PINEAPPLE	:SR		159	89.30	0.40	0.30	9.16	0.30	12.55	2.20	3.10	2.10	0.40	1.40	4.15	—	2.70	—	28.60
CUSTARD APPLE (CHERIMOYA)	CR			89.80	—	—	11.70	1.04	18.40	—	0.81	0.25	—	2.43	1.67	—	2.74	—	26.30
CACTUS FRUIT	::			92.90	1.40	1.30	3.30	2.70	—	—	—	—	—	—	—	—	—	—	—
CACTUS LEAVES	::			94.66	0.70	0.09	8.00	1.23	—	—	—	—	—	—	—	—	—	—	—
GUAVA	::		43	89.50	1.30	0.70	8.05	0.50	15.47	—	0.75	0.48	—	2.44	1.05	0.30	1.55	—	22.04
GUAVA, STRAWBERRY	::			89.47	0.76	0.95	21.66	0.77	—	—	—	—	—	—	—	—	—	—	—
JUJUBE	::			75.96	1.44	0.21	23.70	0.73	—	—	—	—	—	—	—	—	—	—	—
DURIAN	::			70.76	2.30	—	20.00	1.24	—	—	—	—	—	—	—	—	—	—	—
SAPODILLA	::			77.58	0.87	0.55	21.75	1.00	—	—	—	—	—	—	—	—	—	—	—
SAPOTE, WHITE	::			76.36	0.87	0.55	4.40	0.47	—	—	—	—	—	—	—	—	—	—	—
STAR APPLE	::			91.57	2.35	1.38	21.75	0.40	—	—	—	—	—	—	—	—	—	—	—
LITCHI, FRESH	::		43	82.81	1.15	0.20	15.30	0.54	—	—	—	—	—	—	—	—	—	—	—
LITCHI, DRIED	::			16.40	2.90	0.80	78.00	1.90	—	—	—	—	—	—	—	—	—	—	—
TAMARIND	::		132	65.65	1.36	—	31.43	1.56	—	—	—	—	—	—	—	—	—	—	—

ABBREVIATIONS: C = Cosmic   S = Solar   T = Terrestrial   H = Human   A = Animal   R = Radiations

CATEGORY 2

NAMES OF PARTS OF BODY AND OF FOODS	PREDOMINANT RADIATIONS	PREDOMINANT VITAMINS	CALORIES Per 100 Grams	WATER	PROTEIN	FAT	CARBOHYDRATES (SUGAR, STARCH)	MINERAL MATTER	POTASSIUM K_2O	SODIUM Na_2O	CALCIUM CaO	MAGNESIUM MgO	IRON Fe_2O_3	PHOSPHORUS P_2O_5	SULPHUR SO_2	SILICON SiO_2	CHLORINE	FLUORINE	TOTAL
GROUP A	TR-SR	ABCE																	
TOMATO	SR	ABCE	24	94.10	0.90	0.20	3.75	1.05	82.50	32.90	11.35	13.55	1.00	10.75	5.00	1.75	18.00	—	176.80
CUCUMBER	"	"	16	95.96	1.20	0.10	2.30	0.44	41.20	10.00	7.30	4.15	1.40	20.20	6.90	8.00	6.60	—	105.75
GROUP B																			
TURNIP	TR	"	36	83.82	3.50	0.10	11.30	1.28	59.10	7.10	14.24	4.66	0.75	18.27	12.10	1.40	8.30	—	125.92
TURNIP LEAF	SR	"	47	89.53	1.90	—	7.40	1.07	22.63	8.16	27.39	2.78	1.29	3.71	4.38	—	—	—	70.34
RADISH (LARGE)	TR	"	24	94.11	1.20	0.15	3.80	0.74	18.00	3.05	6.60	2.85	1.00	33.70	6.35	6.75	4.00	—	82.30
RADISH (SMALL)	"	"	24	93.00	1.60	0.50	3.80	1.40	35.10	23.15	16.30	3.35	3.00	12.00	7.15	1.00	10.00	—	111.05
PARSNIP	"	"	61	87.50	1.60	0.10	9.70	1.10	33.80	0.32	4.80	2.50	0.25	10.25	8.00	9.60	10.40	—	79.92
BEETROOT	"	"	32	82.40	1.00	0.10	15.80	0.70	38.70	9.00	5.45	2.73	0.26	8.27	6.15	7.90	9.00	—	87.46
SUGAR BEET	"	"	31	88.75	1.91	0.03	8.64	0.70	23.40	3.35	2.30	7.35	0.45	4.60	2.60	—	1.85	—	37.30
SUGAR BEET LEAF	SR	"	28	88.00	1.20	0.20	8.10	0.50	8.45	11.00	15.60	0.10	0.40	3.25	7.35	—	—	—	63.60
BEETROOT, RED	TR	"	44	85.53	4.90	0.20	8.20	0.70	29.30	21.60	2.50	5.65	1.00	1.70	4.45	2.00	2.95	—	41.65
KOHLRABI	SR	"	42	87.50	1.00	0.20	9.40	1.17	25.46	5.40	9.15	3.04	2.50	2.55	13.30	2.05	4.10	—	67.20
CARROT	TR	"	47	93.12	1.70	0.30	3.90	0.90	56.05	14.63	7.00	8.70	0.70	8.83	2.60	1.66	3.18	—	69.75
OXALIS (SORREL)	"	"	32	80.26	1.80	0.14	16.70	0.98	25.32	0.85	7.00	1.55	9.85	21.35	2.70	—	8.70	—	125.80
ARTICHOKE	"	"	75	80.35	1.80	0.10	17.00	1.10	25.32	5.38	1.80	1.60	2.00	7.40	—	5.30	2.06	—	53.36
JERUSALEM ARTICHOKE	"	"	78		1.50			1.05	26.20	5.80			2.15	7.65		—	2.10	—	50.00

35% OF THE DAILY RATION — RAW VEGETABLES — ELIMINATIVE FOODS

IN 1,000 PARTS OF WATER FREE SUBSTANCE

ABBREVIATIONS: C = Cosmic   S = Solar   T = Terrestrial   H = Human   A = Animal   R = Radiations

Food	R	N																
GROUP C																		
LETTUCE	SR	19	95.07	1.40	0.30	2.20	1.03	67.94	13.55	26.56	11.20	9.40	16.62	6.87	14.64	13.82	—	180.60
LETTUCE, ROMAINE	"	19	92.50	1.54	0.43	4.20	1.33	44.90	62.70	21.10	7.60	2.30	19.40	6.90	5.30	7.40	—	177.60
LETTUCE, LAMBS'	"	20	93.41	2.70	0.40	2.70	0.79	53.00	11.20	7.20	2.60	0.45	10.20	5.80	24.00	5.70	—	120.15
BRUSSELS SPROUTS	SR	58	88.03	3.50	0.20	6.80	1.37	31.40	0.35	2.40	2.35	0.60	20.25	35.30	—	2.75	—	95.40
CABBAGE	"	48	91.87	1.90	0.20	4.80	1.23	45.38	11.68	21.65	4.90	0.86	11.07	17.10	—	10.45	—	124.19
CABBAGE, SAVOY	"	32	88.36	3.30	0.70	6.00	1.64	34.80	12.95	27.17	8.13	2.16	18.63	10.41	1.10	10.03	—	130.35
CABBAGE, RED	"	25	91.34	1.83	0.70	5.85	0.77	17.00	9.33	21.49	3.41	0.03	3.00	9.58	6.07	10.51	—	74.77
CAULIFLOWER	"	33	91.82	2.50	0.30	4.55	0.83	40.46	5.34	5.10	3.37	0.91	18.42	11.86	0.38	3.10	—	91.97
OKRA	"	—	90.20	1.60	0.20	7.40	0.60	8.80	12.60	—	3.37	0.01	9.00	7.10	3.37	—	—	61.21
DANDELION	"	—	87.15	2.80	0.70	7.45	1.90	50.95	13.63	25.20	11.00	1.10	10.22	2.68	—	3.47	—	128.52
LEEK BULB	"	42	88.26	2.80	0.30	6.50	1.24	30.70	14.15	10.40	2.90	1.10	16.70	7.40	9.17	3.10	—	100.35
LEEK LEAF	"	50	92.21	1.50	0.30	5.10	0.69	33.25	5.55	17.70	3.60	7.60	6.25	3.35	7.40	5.50	—	75.70
ASPARAGUS	"	23	94.81	1.80	0.25	2.60	0.54	20.94	14.77	9.33	3.72	0.50	16.07	5.35	9.50	5.10	—	87.69
SWISS CHARD	"	—	92.50	1.54	0.43	4.20	1.33	44.90	62.70	21.70	7.60	2.94	19.40	6.90	5.30	7.40	—	178.20
GROUP D																		
CELERY	TR	18	94.50	1.10	0.10	3.30	1.00	48.60	65.25	14.70	6.75	1.60	14.50	6.50	4.30	17.80	—	180.00
CELERY ROOT	SR	18	85.46	1.50	0.40	11.80	0.84	22.70	—	6.90	3.05	0.75	6.75	2.95	2.10	8.45	—	53.65
SPINACH	TR	32	89.36	3.50	0.60	4.44	2.10	29.90	63.90	21.50	11.50	6.05	18.05	12.45	8.10	11.30	—	182.75
WATERCRESS	SR	27	95.24	0.80	0.10	1.30	1.46	49.75	17.25	35.00	8.60	0.35	22.40	53.90	—	7.75	—	190.00
CHICORY ROOT	TR	20	79.97	1.10	0.20	18.30	0.73	13.20	5.05	2.40	1.60	0.85	4.30	2.70	—	2.75	—	32.85
GREEN PEPPER	SR	—	93.20	4.30	0.10	4.60	1.00	—	—	—	—	—	—	—	—	—	—	—
SALSIFY	TR	75	87.40	—	0.50	17.10	1.20	—	—	—	—	—	—	—	—	—	—	—
SALSIFY (BLACK)	SR	—	80.40	1.90	0.10	3.00	1.58	15.30	6.40	3.40	2.07	1.48	12.95	5.60	—	1.60	—	48.80
KALE	"	56	93.42	1.90	0.20	8.50	1.10	81.50	5.35	28.10	7.30	1.30	35.50	86.00	—	10.50	—	255.55
RUTABAGA	"	—	88.90	1.30	0.20	8.50	1.10	46.30	13.60	8.80	5.20	1.70	18.10	5.30	—	1.00	—	100.00
GROUP E																		
COW'S MILK, FRESH RAW	SAR	67	87.16	3.55	3.70	4.88	0.71	13.70	5.34	12.24	1.69	0.30	15.79	0.17	0.02	8.04	—	57.29
GOAT'S MILK, FRESH RAW	"	71	87.00	4.30	4.50	4.40	0.80	15.60	3.45	13.90	2.30	0.60	21.05	0.30	0.20	13.50	—	70.90
SHEEP'S MILK, FRESH RAW	"	107	80.80	6.50	6.90	4.90	0.90	14.00	4.65	11.70	2.15	0.17	17.70	0.20	0.10	5.70	—	47.40
BUTTERMILK	"	35	91.00	3.00	0.50	4.80	0.70	18.10	8.50	14.40	2.60	0.60	21.80	1.30	—	9.70	—	77.00
SKIM-MILK	"	35	90.50	3.40	0.30	5.10	0.70	22.60	7.10	15.20	2.20	0.60	13.40	2.40	—	10.20	—	73.70
WHEY	"	32	93.79	0.60	0.07	5.10	0.44	21.85	9.75	13.65	0.25	0.40	12.00	1.90	—	11.20	—	71.00

1.5% OF THE DAILY RATION — CONDIMENTS WITH OIL AND LEMON JUICE FOR SALADS

Food	R	N																
GROUP F																		
CHIVE	TR	—	85.75	2.80	0.50	10.00	0.95	18.05	2.28	11.27	2.90	0.80	8.12	6.66	8.10	2.32	—	52.40
ONION	"	49	87.60	1.60	0.10	9.90	0.60	12.10	1.55	10.65	2.55	2.20	7.25	2.65	—	1.35	—	48.40
GARLIC	SR	142	63.70	6.80	0.10	27.90	1.50	28.70	12.65	31.95	11.55	1.00	20.30	20.05	2.40	—	—	—
DILL		—	85.90	3.50	0.70	7.30	2.40	—	—	—	—	—	—	—	—	—	—	—
PARSLEY	SR	70	86.45	3.70	0.90	7.45	1.50	—	—	—	—	—	—	—	—	14.75	—	143.35
HORSERADISH	TR	—	79.45	2.70	0.35	16.00	1.50	19.81	2.57	5.28	1.87	1.25	4.96	19.84	8.18	8.18	—	71.94

ABBREVIATIONS: C = Cosmic   S = Solar   T = Terrestrial   H = Human   A = Animal   R = Radiations

COMPOSITION OF MINERAL MATTER IN 1,000 PARTS OF WATER FREE SUBSTANCE

10% OF THE DAILY RATION — CEREALS AND STARCHES — RECONSTRUCTIVE FOODS

NAMES OF PARTS OF BODY AND OF FOODS	PRED. RADIATIONS	PRED. VITAMINS	CALORIES Per 100 Grams	WATER	PROTEIN	FAT	CARBOHYDRATES (SUGAR, STARCH)	MINERAL MATTER	POTASSIUM K_2O	SODIUM Na_2O	CALCIUM CaO	MAGNESIUM MgO	IRON Fe_2O_3	PHOSPHORUS P_2O_2	SULPHUR SO_2	SILICON SiO_2	CHLORINE	FLUORINE	TOTAL
CATEGORY 3	SR	BE																	
GROUP A																			
BANANA	CR	:	99	75.30	1.30	0.60	22.00	0.80	16.10	5.60	0.68	2.40	0.07	2.85	1.20	0.80	2.70	—	32.40
POTATO	TR	:	95	75.67	2.08	0.15	21.00	1.10	26.56	1.33	1.15	2.18	0.48	7.47	2.89	0.88	1.55	—	44.49
SWEET POTATO		:	—	69.00	1.80	0.70	27.40	1.10	18.60	2.20	3.10	0.85	0.50	2.20	1.05	1.40	5.50	—	35.40
BREADFRUIT	:CR	:	—	82.17	1.57	0.51	14.60	1.15	17.50	2.10	6.30	0.50	0.01	5.10	3.75	—	1.50	—	36.76
GROUP B																			
WHEAT, WHOLE	SR	:	352	13.40	13.60	1.90	69.10	2.00	7.20	0.50	0.75	2.80	0.30	10.90	0.09	0.46	0.07	—	23.07
WHEAT, GERM OF		:	379	12.30	35.70	13.10	31.20	5.70	15.15	0.33	—	9.35	0.38	27.80	0.13	0.50	—	—	55.29
WHEAT, BRAN		:	323	12.95	16.60	3.50	62.10	4.85	4.15	4.10	1.65	1.05	0.30	4.75	0.60	—	6.80	—	23.30
WHEAT BREAD, WHOLE		:	251	35.70	8.90	1.80	52.10	1.50	2.35	6.40	1.55	2.35	0.45	4.50	0.85	—	4.80	—	23.20
PUMPERNICKEL BREAD		:	223	50.45	4.20	0.70	43.30	1.35	5.60	2.70	1.50	1.20	0.08	5.85	2.90	—	1.90	—	21.23
SWEDISH RYE CRISP		:	370	18.45	8.00	0.60	70.10	1.95			1.00								
GERMINATED WHEAT GRAIN—		:																	
WHOLE		:																	
CRUSHED		:																	
SUN-BAKED		:																	
OVEN-BAKED																			
BOILED			352	13.40	13.60	1.90	69.10	2.00	7.20	0.50	0.75	2.80	0.30	10.90	0.09	0.46	0.07	—	23.07

(Average figures. Exact figures depend on proportion of water used)

GROUP C

Food	370	17.09	11.50	1.80	67.80	1.81	6.84	0.31	0.61	2.39	0.25	10.16	0.28	0.30	0.01	—	21.15
RYE, WHOLE	343	15.54	9.85	4.60	68.50	1.51	5.50	0.20	0.36	2.87	0.15	8.44	0.15	0.39	0.35	—	18.41
CORN, WHOLE YELLOW (MAIZE)	—	75.90	3.10	1.10	19.20	0.70	8.50	3.20	0.50	2.65	0.07	8.28	3.68	0.50	1.12	—	28.50
CORN, GREEN (MAIZE)	363	5.70	10.70	5.00	77.30	1.30	3.60	0.67	0.59	1.78	0.22	8.60	0.10	0.40	0.02	—	15.98
CORN, POPPED	350	13.87	7.85	0.88	76.50	1.00	6.00	—	1.35	9.15	4.00	22.85	0.12	8.85	—	—	52.30
RICE, WHOLE	—	14.40	11.10	3.80	62.10	4.55	4.46	0.71	0.28	3.26	0.42	13.00	—	1.60	0.35	—	23.73
RICE, BRAN	355	15.00	9.00	7.85	70.25	1.95	6.00	1.35	2.25	4.25	0.40	14.30	0.80	0.40	0.60	—	34.50
MILLET	410	23.58	10.40	5.20	57.80	3.02	10.40	1.30	1.50	2.10	0.60	7.15	1.45	0.20	1.10	—	21.40
OATS, WHOLE	410	7.70	16.70	7.30	66.20	2.10	6.50	1.00	1.10	1.75	0.05	8.10	0.55	0.20	0.35	—	20.20
OATS, ROLLED	380	7.30	16.05	7.20	67.50	1.95	5.50	1.68	1.21	3.41	0.47	13.35	0.70	0.06	1.10	—	27.40
OATMEAL	343	14.74	11.41	2.68	68.79	2.38	6.32	1.05	1.10	3.70	0.40	15.00	—	0.20	0.35	—	31.30
BUCK WHEAT	339	19.10	11.10	2.20	64.90	2.70	8.80	—	—	—	—	—	—	—	—	—	—
BARLEY, WHOLE	—	—	—	—	—	—	—	—	—	—	—	—	—	—	—	—	—

GROUP D

Food																	
SORGHUM	346	15.40	9.10	3.60	69.80	2.10	6.00	0.90	0.35	5.20	0.58	10.60	0.12	—	0.25	—	24.00
SAGO (TR)	—	12.20	9.00	0.40	78.10	0.30	—	—	—	—	—	—	—	—	—	—	—
TAPIOCA	350	11.40	1.80	0.10	88.00	0.10	—	—	—	—	—	—	—	—	—	—	—
TARO	100	73.00	1.80	0.20	23.20	1.20	—	—	—	—	—	—	—	—	—	—	—
YAM	100	73.80	1.10	0.20	23.30	0.90	—	—	—	—	—	—	—	—	—	—	—
CASSAVA, SWEET	100	67.80	—	0.20	30.20	0.70	—	—	—	—	—	—	—	—	—	—	—

ABBREVIATIONS: C = Cosmic   S = Solar   T = Terrestrial   H = Human   A = Animal   R = Radiations

NAMES OF PARTS OF BODY AND OF FOODS	PREDOMINANT RADIATIONS (CR-AR)	PREDOMINANT VITAMINS (ABD)	CALORIES Per 100 Grams	WATER	PROTEIN	FAT	CARBOHYDRATES (SUGAR, STARCH)	MINERAL MATTER	POTASSIUM K_2O	SODIUM Na_2O	CALCIUM CaO	MAGNESIUM MgO	IRON Fe_2O_3	PHOSPHORUS P_2O_5	SULPHUR SO_2	SILICON SiO_2	CHLORINE	FLUORINE	TOTAL
CATEGORY 4								5% OF THE DAILY RATION – DRIED, SWEET AND OILY FRUITS AND ANIMAL PRODUCTS – STRONGLY RECONSTRUCTIVE FOODS											
GROUP A																			
RAISIN	CR	..	296	17.10	2.60	3.30	73.60	3.40	19.40	3.30	2.45	2.30	0.60	7.30	2.55	—	2.10	—	40.00
PRUNE	..	..	302	24.40	2.10	—	71.20	2.30	19.15	0.80	1.40	1.75	0.60	4.20	0.80	0.90	0.10	—	29.18
FIG, DRIED (SMYRNA)	..	..	276	18.80	4.30	0.30	74.20	2.40	17.10	0.90	3.30	1.68	0.66	3.85	1.20	—	0.61	—	29.30
FIG, DRIED (BLACK)	..	..	276	27.30	5.50	1.00	63.00	3.20	10.50	9.60	3.50	3.40	0.60	6.30	2.70	2.40	1.00	—	40.00
DATE	..	..	308	23.50	2.10	2.80	70.00	1.60	10.50	1.00	1.15	1.19	0.06	1.00	1.20	—	3.90	—	20.00
APPLE, DRIED	..	..	250	33.20	1.60	2.00	62.00	1.00	—	—	—	—	—	—	—	—	—	—	—
APRICOT, DRIED	..	..	225	29.40	4.70	1.00	62.50	2.00	—	—	—	—	—	—	—	—	—	—	—
PEAR, DRIED	..	..	252	23.40	2.80	5.40	66.00	2.40	—	—	—	—	—	—	—	—	—	—	—
PEACH, DRIED	..	..	254	24.25	3.15	0.45	50.00	2.15	—	—	—	—	—	—	—	—	—	—	—
CURRANT, DRIED (ZANTE)	..	..	180	17.20	2.40	1.70	74.20	4.50	30.00	3.15	1.60	1.85	0.30	12.40	3.10	—	1.75	—	54.15
GROUP B																			
HONEY	CSAR	..	321	18.20	0.40	—	81.20	0.20	0.02	0.10	2.35	0.01	0.12	0.18	0.01	—	0.01	—	2.80
SUGAR CANE	SR	..	100	75.43	1.50	0.55	21.82	0.70	—	—	—	—	—	—	—	—	—	—	28.40
RAW SUGAR	STR	..	350	4.14	0.30	—	94.60	0.96	5.97	1.30	0.70	0.03	0.04	0.03	0.95	—	0.78	—	9.80
MOLASSES	SR	..	246	25.10	2.40	—	69.30	3.20	27.00	0.38	4.22	1.36	0.02	0.88	2.58	—	6.34	—	42.78

Food	Type	1	2	3	4	5	6	7	8	9	10	11	12	13	14	15	16	17
GROUP C																		
ALMOND	CR	639	4.90	21.40	54.40	16.80	5.23	2.50	0.38	3.04	3.95	0.23	10.10	0.96	0.04	0.06	—	23.99
WALNUT, ENGLISH	"	754	2.50	18.40	64.40	13.00	2.20	1.70	0.17	0.97	2.88	0.61	10.10	0.22	0.12	0.12	—	17.39
WALNUT, BLACK	"	731	2.50	27.60	56.30	11.70		1.90									—	34.60
BRAZIL NUT	"	742	8.60	17.40	65.00	5.70	6.65	3.30	0.37	6.10	2.90	0.10	13.30	4.33		0.85	—	16.67
PECAN	"		7.10	12.10	70.70	8.50	5.80	1.60	0.36	1.33	2.20	0.23	6.75				—	
BUTTERNUT	"		4.50	27.90	61.20	3.40		3.00									—	
PARADISE NUT	"		2.30	22.20	62.60	10.20		2.70									—	
CANDLENUT	"	620	8.67	21.40	61.70	4.90	11.40	2.30	0.28	1.07	1.87	0.14	5.50	3.00	0.04	0.01	—	23.31
CHESTNUT, DRIED	"	194	5.90	10.70		74.20	12.30	2.20	0.01	0.90	0.15	0.01	5.10	0.45		0.15	—	19.07
WATER CHESTNUT	"	500	42.93	4.00	1.20	50.00	9.75	1.77	1.30	1.10	1.30	0.40	4.80	0.85		3.20	—	22.70
COCOANUT	"	600	14.10	5.70	50.60	27.90		1.30									—	
COCOANUT, DRIED	"		3.50	6.30	57.40	31.50		0.80									—	
COCOANUT MILK	"	4	92.70	0.40	1.50	4.60		3.86									—	
PIGNOLIA, ITALIAN	"		6.20	33.90	48.20	7.90		2.10									—	
PISTACHIO	"	700	4.20	22.60	54.50	15.60	7.20	2.90	2.18	7.73	5.94	0.42	12.81	1.03	1.13	1.03	—	39.47
HICKORY NUT	"		3.70	15.40	67.40	11.40	5.70	2.40	0.75	2.62	4.20	0.60	13.15	4.46			—	27.02
BEECH NUT	"	617	12.74	21.70	42.50	19.20	6.65	2.25	0.20	3.60	1.98	0.46	7.30	0.45	0.05	0.60	—	25.05
PINON	"	636	3.30	14.60	61.90	17.30	9.27	2.20	0.21	0.95	2.29	0.27	10.60			0.23	—	24.32
FILBERT	SR	554	5.40	16.50	61.60	11.70		3.00									—	
PEANUT	"	930	9.75	29.80	43.50	14.70		2.50									—	
PEANUT BUTTER	CR	930	4.90	29.30	46.50	17.10	12.96	1.35	0.82	1.95	4.00	0.02	13.95	1.25	0.55	0.30	—	35.80
ALMOND BUTTER	"		2.20	5.70	61.50	11.60	11.75	2.34	8.35	2.15	2.36	0.67	8.00	5.05	0.22	6.45	—	45.00
CAROB (ST. JOHN'S BREAD)	SR	490	23.70	12.00	1.10	67.00	27.02	3.50	2.52	2.50	0.06	0.30	0.46	0.36	0.22	0.06	—	33.50
COCOA BEAN	CR		8.80	2.10	49.30	6.00	6.12	7.42	2.80	2.87	4.65	0.60	13.38	0.87	5.54	0.90	—	37.73
AVOCADO	SR		70.55	5.24	20.00	10.45											—	
OLIVE, DRIED	"		30.07	14.20	51.90	14.50											—	
SUNFLOWER SEED	SR		10.50	35.99	32.30												—	
SESAME	"	381	9.14		24.62	22.83											—	
GROUP D																		
COTTAGE CHEESE	SAR	192	72.55	20.90	1.00	4.30	5.40	1.25	0.90	14.35	1.00	0.30	15.35	0.60		7.10	—	45.00
CREAM	"	245	74.00	2.50	18.50	4.50	5.15	0.50	1.55	4.25	0.60	0.50	3.90	0.45		2.00	—	18.40
BUTTER, COW'S	"	752	11.00	1.00	85.00		1.75	3.00	12.10	0.96	0.18	0.05	0.12	6.85		11.75	—	33.70
EGG, WHOLE	"	171	73.70	12.55	12.10	0.55	6.27	1.10	9.56	4.56	0.46	0.17	15.72	0.13	0.13	3.72	—	40.22
EGG, WHITE	"	50	85.75	12.70	0.25	0.70	13.21	0.60	13.30	1.18	1.18	0.25	1.85	0.88	0.45	12.08	—	44.38
EGG, YOLK	"	381	50.65	16.20	31.95	0.10	2.70	1.10	1.44	3.17	0.51	0.40	15.22		0.21	0.45	—	24.10

ABBREVIATIONS: C = Cosmic   S = Solar   T = Terrestrial   H = Human   A = Animal   R = Radiations

CATEGORY 5

35, 15 and 10% OF THE DAILY RATION – COOKED VEGETABLES – CONSTRUCTIVE FOODS
(Permissible once or twice a week but not recommended)

Names of parts of body and of foods	Pred. Radiations	Pred. Vitamins	Calories per 100 g	Water	Protein	Fat	Carbohydrates (sugar, starch)	Mineral matter	K_2O	Na_2O	CaO	MgO	Fe_2O_3	P_2O_5	SO_2	SiO_2	Chlorine	Fluorine	Total
GROUP A (35%) — All Vegetables of Category II in cooked form, and the following:	SR	B																	
PUMPKIN	:	:	25	91.47	1.10	0.13	6.50	0.70	13.85	15.22	5.55	2.45	1.88	23.80	1.73	5.27	0.30	—	70.05
LIMA BEAN, GREEN	:	:	32	68.90	7.10	0.70	22.00	1.70	33.90	4.75	1.40	3.60	0.14	6.60	3.10	—	0.50	—	53.99
KIDNEY BEAN, GREEN	:	:	132	86.90	3.90	0.20	8.30	0.70	23.30	1.70	2.75	1.65	0.05	5.65	7.00	—	1.90	—	44.00
STRING BEAN, FRESH	:	:	40	86.40	3.90	0.20	8.30	1.20	32.00	1.75	7.50	6.25	0.05	6.50	12.75	—	7.10	—	73.80
PEAS, GREEN	:	:	90	74.60	7.00	0.50	16.90	1.00	15.40	1.10	1.60	2.80	0.04	11.20	6.00	—	1.40	—	39.54
GROUP B (15%)																			
EGG-PLANT	:	:	28	92.50	1.20	0.30	5.10	0.50	39.05	2.80	3.05	4.20	0.25	9.50	4.45	—	6.70	—	70.00
SOYA BEAN	:	:	442	10.75	34.00	16.80	33.70	4.75	24.65	0.60	3.45	3.45	0.28	17.50	2.65	0.27	0.40	—	53.25
LENTIL	TR	:	337	16.06	25.70	1.90	53.30	3.04	11.60	4.60	2.10	0.90	0.60	12.20	1.20	0.65	1.50	—	34.70
MUSHROOM	:	:	28	90.30	2.60	0.30	6.10	0.70	32.68	1.05	0.65	2.18	1.02	21.60	2.50	1.05	0.57	—	62.90
CHAMPIGNON	:	:	39	92.11	3.74	0.15	3.50	0.50	37.87	1.27	0.55	0.37	0.85	11.50	18.15	0.20	3.45	—	75.06
TRUFFLE	:	:	93	83.28	7.70	0.50	6.60	1.92	31.50	1.50	8.15	1.05	4.65	27.65	5.00	—	1.10	—	80.80
GROUP C (10%)	SR	:																	
BEAN, DRIED	:	:	332	21.84	24.30	1.60	49.00	3.26	15.85	0.42	1.91	2.73	0.19	14.86	1.30	0.25	0.69	—	38.20
BEAN, BLACKEYE	:	:	338	11.23	21.43	1.28	61.28	4.78	—	—	—	—	—	—	—	—	—	—	—
HORSE-BEAN	:	:	342	28.25	18.00	0.50	50.50	2.75	15.25	0.40	0.15	0.30	0.10	14.30	1.15	—	0.60	—	32.25
LIMA BEAN, DRIED	:	:	334	10.40	18.10	1.50	65.90	4.10	27.60	4.10	1.25	3.10	0.01	6.10	2.60	—	0.04	—	44.80
KIDNEY BEAN, DRIED	:	:	336	17.44	23.12	2.28	53.63	3.53	18.00	0.58	2.60	3.00	0.13	14.30	1.65	0.23	0.34	—	40.83
PEAS, DRIED	:	:	334	20.37	22.85	1.80	52.40	2.58	13.06	0.30	1.45	2.42	0.24	10.87	1.03	1.27	0.53	—	31.17
COW PEAS, DRIED	:	:	348	13.00	21.40	1.40	60.80	3.40	21.00	2.40	1.50	3.15	—	6.85	3.60	—	0.60	—	39.10
CHICK PEAS (GARBANZAS)	:	:	323	30.24	13.00	1.60	51.50	3.76	8.10	4.00	1.45	18.35	0.80	13.10	1.10	—	0.95	—	44.25

ABBREVIATIONS: C = Cosmic   S = Solar   T = Terrestrial   H = Human   A = Animal   R = Radiations

9

TRIDOSHA

Serious students of nutrition can benefit from a knowledge of Tridosha which is the basis for the Hindu concept of medicine and diet.

According to the theory of Tridosha, man is composed of three primordial cosmic elements — air, fire, and water. In modern nuclear physics these three elements are known as neutron, electron, and proton. The macrocosm consists of three cosmic elements. Man, being a little world, or microcosm, is also a combination and reflection of these three primeval elements. When these elements are in balance and in harmony within the individual, they create and maintain health. When they become out of balance and are in disharmony with natural changes taking place in the macrocosm, the individual loses equilibrium and the resulting disharmony tends to encourage disease. The symptoms of the disease produced are only an outward manifestation of the underlying disharmony, disorder and imbalance. To cure the symptoms, a new equilibrium must be acquired, or another set of symptoms will arise to portray a new disharmony.

Disharmony is indicated by changes in the patient's pulse. Like the whole man, the pulse is understood in terms of the three primal elements. The physician will not only study the pulse's speed and regularity, as physicians do in the West, but also its rhythm and the proportion of one primal element to another. There are three layers of pulse which can be felt by applying three degrees of pressure: superficial, medium and deep pressure.

Air is called *Vat* or *Vayu* in Hindu medical philosophy and science. It stands for vital power and is the first principle of life. In the individual its chief reticulum is the autonomic nervous system. Air is of great assistance to the elements of fire and water and has a high mixing quality. In modern language it is the neutron which splits up atoms into electrons and protons. When it joins with electrons atomic heat is produced. Conversely, atomic cold is produced when it joins with protons.

Characteristics are speed: talks fast, eats fast, walks fast. Time: Afternoon. Rains. Age 40 years and beyond. A pulse predominated by air moves like a serpent, like an eel, and is crooked.

Fire is called *Pit*. It is manifested in the human body as heat, and is conveyed by the circulatory system. It is a lame element and cannot move without air as a driving force. Fire is the electron. Therefore, when it joins with neutrons it produces atomic heat.

Characteristics: Hot, flashy, intelligent, irritable, vigorous. Time: Noon. Autumn. Age: 16-40 years.

A fire pulse is indicated by a jumpy, froglike, or birdlike movement.

Water is called *Kaj* or *Kapha*. It is the ruler of all the mucous membranes and maintains the integrity of the body. Water keeps fire in check. It also is a lame element and needs air as a moving force. Water is proton. When it mixes with neutron it produces atomic cold.

Characteristics: Lubricating, self-controlled, mild, stable, patient. Time: Morning. Spring. Age: 1-16 years.

A water pulse is elegant, swanlike, pigeonlike, and slow moving.

During the process of eating food, the heat contained within the fire is generated by the movement of air as pacified by water. The water is moved by air and ameliorates any excess of fire. All three elements combine to mix the food from the mouth into the oesophagus and on into the stomach. It is then divided into liquids and solids. The liquid is eliminated by the kidneys. The solids are mixed with bile, itself a mixture of the three primary elements made in the liver. The food mixed with bile is then absorbed into the system to support the liver and the blood. The waste matter from this process passes further on into the colon and is then eliminated.

Air always plays the vital role of being the moving force. It moves the essence of the food and then moves the blood. In the elimination process it moves the urinary liquids and the waste material in the bowel towards the rectum. Water, on the other hand, plays a passive role, controlled by air and fire. In return, it controls the fire. Fire helps maintain the heat of the body and relates it to the atmosphere. Thus it keeps the body in a state of survival during cold by heating it. During heat it allows itself to be cooled. Fire is pacified by both air and water.

Therefore, foods that are pacified by air and water are essentially fire. Foods that are pacified by air and fire are water. And foods that are pacified by water are both air and fire.

It has been proved that each intake of food lasts for five days and nights. When the heat of the fire is pacified by air and water there is a resulting mild glow of warmth in the body. This warmth produces life and gives pleasure, strength and form to the body. A person's system may become over-heated as a result of excess air and fire. Thus an unbalanced combination or interaction of the three elements will reduce light (*Ojas*). In turn, the rhythm of life is reduced, elimination of bodily solids and liquids diminishes, the body becomes congested and disease arises.

The same elemental process can be seen at work in a field where our food grows. Water falls to the field from above or is carried by an arterial irrigation system of various pumps, canals and channels. It is kept moving by winds and breezes — air — and is thereby distributed to various parts of the field. The water and air go to the roots of the plant beneath the earth, and the earth's drainage allows the excess to be filtered away and redistributed. The roots of the plant are protected by the elements within the earth and are kept warm through solar energy. Thus the natural elemental process keeps the plant alive.

Those foods that grow in excess of water such as rice, barley, cucumber, marrow, etc., are water foods. Fruits, nuts and flower seeds, such as those of the sunflower, which absorb heat, are fire foods and are likely to contain fat. Lentils, pulses, wheat, barley and millet can retain heat because of their tough pods and therefore are classified as air or protein foods. Root foods such as carrots, potatoes, and turnips are a combination of heat and water and therefore contain a balance of fire and water.

It is in the growth of these foods and fruits that one can begin to observe the expression of their predominant factors. Although no particular food is in essence solely air, fire, or water, it is thought of in terms of its major prevailing element.

In considering the diet of a sick person, one must decide what the patient's predominant needs are at each mealtime. The physician would make this choice in accordance with the pulse. There would be no point in giving fire foods in hot weather, in fever, or when the person is in a state of great aggravation or temper. In such a case the pulse would indicate too much fire. After considering the relationship of air and water to the excess of fire, the appropriate food could then be chosen. For example, in a high fever with plenty of sweat, I would tend to choose air foods such as apples, bananas, corn or oatmeal. On the other hand, in a high fever with thirst and no sweat I would use more water foods such as lemons, grapefruits or pears. And in high fever with no sweat but with dryness and thirst, I would use air and water foods such as yogurt, milk, endive, beetroots, grapes, etc.

Tridosha is an all-embracing theory which concerns itself with all internal and external conditions as created by the three cosmic elements: Air, Fire, and Water. It has been known and practised in India for at least 3,000 years and is an invaluable contribution to World Knowledge.

Ayurvedic Tridosha

POSITIVE

FIRE — PIT — COSMIC — ELECTRONS — RED — HOT
Characteristics: Blood. Oxygenoid. Above and inside of body. Noon. Autumn. Anti-lameness. Fast. Movement of a sparrow, a crow, a frog — forward jumping jerks.
Residence: Blood. Sweat. Chyle. Watery part of muscles. Duodenum.
Residence (Chinese opinion): Liver. Spleen. Heart. Eyes. Skin. Duodenum.
Pulses: *Pachaka:* Digestion. Chyle. Faeces. Sweat. *Ranjaka:* Colour. Chyle. Liver. Spleen. *Sadhaka:* Fulfilment. Reduces Delusion. Increases intellect and memory related to true heart. *Alochka:* Seeing. Pupil of the eye. *Bhraka:* Elasticity and shine of skin.
Worse: Exposure to sun. Fire. Summer. Autumn. Moon. Midnight. Anger. Fear. Grief. Exertion. Indigestion. Unnatural sexual appetites. Two hours after foods. Honey. Bitter foods. Acids. Salts. Fish. Meat. Mutton. Wines. Curds. Wheys.
Purifier: Sweet. Bitter. Astringents. Mainly cereals. Leguminous plants and beans.
Pacifier: Carbohydrates.

NEUTRAL ZONE

AIR — VAYU — NEUTRONS — BLUE
Characteristics: Nerve force. Hydrogenoid. Light. Cold. Dry. Mobile. Piercing. Anti-sycotic. Movement. Thinking. Seeing. Hearing. Foetal expulsion. Snakelike rolling fast movement.
Residence: Intestines (esp. lower intestine). Thighs. Loins. Feet. Bones.
Pulses: *Prana:* Mouth. Protects the heart. *Udana:* Upwards. Speech. Cough. Sneeze. *Samona:* Even. Splits food into fragments. Separates waste matter. *Vyana:* Diffused. Serum supply. Bleeding. Perspiration.

Apana: Downward. Expels foetus, excretions.
Worse: Clouds. Storms. Rain. Afternoon 2-6p.m. 2.6a.m. 4 hours after meals.
Purifier: Enema. Bee and its products. Emetics. Ghee (butter).
Pacifier: Sweet. Sour. Salt.

NEGATIVE

WATER — EARTH — PROTONS — WHITE
Characteristics: Earth. Cold. Carbo-nitrogenoids. Downwards and outside. Lame. Slow. Pigeonlike, peacock, swan or cocklike movement.
Residence: All mucous surfaces of the body. Phlegm. Water. Chest. Stomach. Head. Throat. Joints. Fat.
Pulses: *Kledaka:* Moistener. Stomach. Helps digestion with moistening. *Avalambaka:* Supporter. All the joints. Heart function. *Bodhake:* Feeler. Throat and root of tongue. Imparts taste. *Tarpaka:* Pleasing. Eyes ears nose. *Slesmaka:* Phlegm. Integration of the joints or the grease thereof.
Worse: Winter. Spring. Morning. Evening. 6-10p.m. 2 hours after meals. Day sleep. Sweet. Saline. Sour foods. Carbohydrates. Wine. Butter. Excess of curds. Ices. Cakes. Milk. Sugar. Molasses. Meat. Fish.
Better: Hot pungent foods. Bitter. Astringent. Dry. Late hours of night. Hot baths and exercise. *Best* — Honey.
Purifier: Honey.
Pacifier: Water. Vegetables in leaf.

After studying these descriptions of the three elements, you should be able to identify your type, and will then be able to use the Tridosha of Foods table which follows to guide your choice of diet. For example, if you decide you are a water person, then try to add a few more items of air and fire at each meal to restore the balance. Never eat only one type of food as this would cause an imbalance.

NOTE: A purifying food improves the state of the body and mind. A pacifying food calms down already existing conflicts and tensions.

Tridosha of Foods

Food	Elements	Food	Elements
Apples	Air	Liquids	Air
Artichoke	Water	Meat	Water
Avocado	Water	Milk (fresh)	Air. Fire. Water
Banana	Air. Water	Mint	Fire
Beets	Air. Water	Mushrooms	Water
Biscuits	Air	Nutmeg	Air
Black Olives	Air. Water	Oatmeal	Air. Water
Bottled milk	Water	Onions	Fire
Broccoli	Air	Parsley	Air
Cabbage	Water	Parsnips	Fire
Carrots	Air. Water	Peanuts	Fire
Cauliflower	Water	Pears	Water
Celery	Fire	Peas	Fire
Chestnuts	Air. Water	Pepper (black)	Air. Fire. Water
Chocolate	Fire	Persimmons	Water
Cloves	Fire	Pickles	Fire
Coffee	Fire	Potatoes	Fire
Condiments	Fire	Pulses	Fire
Corn Flakes	Air	Raw sugar	Fire
Corn meal	Air	Rice	Water
Cream	Air. Fire. Water	Salt	Air
Cream cheese	Air. Water	Solids	Fire
Curds	Fire	Soya beans	Fire
Dandelion	Water	Spinach	Water
Dates	Air. Water	Squash	Air
Eggs	Air. Water	Sunflower seed	Fire
Endive	Fire. Water	Sweets	Air. Fire
Escarol	Water	Swiss chard	Water
Fish (fresh)	Air. Fire. Water	Tea	Air
Grapefruit	Water	Tomatoes	Water
Grapes	Air. Water	Turnips	Water
Honey	Water	Vegetables	Water
Kelp	Water	Vinegar	Fire
Kohlrabi	Water	Walnuts	Fire
Lemons	Air	Wheat	Fire
Lettuce	Water	Yellow corn	Air. Water

10

EXERCISE – ALEXANDER TECHNIQUE AND YOGA

Exercise should be regarded as one of the essential inputs of the body and not as a supplementary activity, additional to daily life. Obviously those who earn their livings in the world of sport or dance have a necessity for controlled exercise under specialized guidance, as a part of their professional life. For the rest of us, strenuous physical exercise undertaken on one's own initiative may be inadvisable.

Exercise of a remedial nature is only needed when it serves to correct an imbalance created in other areas of one's life. If one's daily life entails unhealthy habits, a poor working environment, bad eating, forced inactivity, one cannot simply compensate by a strenuous session of sport or an hours dance class. Exercise cannot make up what is lost in daily life.

Ideally exercise should be seen as something one is engaged in at all times. It is a process of one's whole life and should be seen as meeting the physiological needs of the body. Walking, eating, breathing, sleeping, seeing, hearing are all part of the overall process of exercising the body.

Under the guidance of a physician exercise can improve a range of disorders such as high blood-pressure, bad digestion and constipation, depression; if one wishes to engage in exercise for pleasure it is better to choose something such as swimming which serves most of the muscular systems of the body, or walking. Exercise more gently for longer as this serves to improve the circulation and uses the heart more, and avoid bursts of strenuous activity. Do not go to an exercise class because you have failed to exercise in everyday life, rather take the stairs instead of the lift, walk part of the way to work. However, it should be remembered that cycling to work in town or walking in heavy traffic does not constitute healthy exercise.

Walking with awareness can be an experience in physical, mental and emotional renewal. Choose somewhere to walk where you can

observe and enjoy nature, think of the symbiotic relationship one
has with plants and trees and try to breathe being aware of the vital
elements entering the body through the medium of the air.

One thing we must all look for at some point in our daily life is
stillness; our bodies are in motion at some level at all times and a
balance between stillness and movement is part of the harmonious
relationship of the body which is the basis for health.

Alexander Technique

Exercise is not effective as a means of changing bodily habits as we
will naturally exercise in our own individual way which may very
likely be faulty. Alexander Technique is *not* exercise and avoids the
forcible alteration of behaviour patterns. It is the 'right use of the
body' in our daily activities. It is an opportunity to correct bad habits
which have become so familiar they feel 'right'.

F. Mathias Alexander was born in Tasmania in 1869 and trained
as an actor. When his career was jeopardized by problems with his
voice he began to look for the causes in his own posture and habits;
almost by accident he made the astonishing discoveries which led
to the development of what is now known as the Alexander
Technique. He began giving lessons in his methods in 1894 and ten
years later he moved to England where he lived almost continually
until his death in 1955. In 1930 he founded a training school for
teachers of the technique, which became his main work for the rest
of his life; he also wrote several books, including *The Use of the Self*
(1932).

Since our habits of living — posture, movement etc. — are so
ingrained it can take a long time to change these. First it is necessary
to observe what is happening to our bodies daily. What are the causes
of physical discomfort, why do we do things in a certain way? From
here we can gradually help to correct our habits without imposing
an outside force; change must slowly be guided from within with
the help of a teacher. 'The pupil is put through simple movements
which are part of his ordinary life, such as sitting down and standing
up, walking, picking things from the floor, and especially actions
required in his daily occupation. The teacher guides him with his
hands so that he can get the feel of these actions in a way involving
no undue tensions and with good bodily poise. Then with repetitions
at gradually increasing intervals, he begins to maintain this state for
himself and eventually lives in it. When this point is reached he will
be using his body so well that every action he performs will in itself

be a kind of exercise but will have become natural to him.' (From *Maintaining Nature's Safety Margin by the Alexander Method*, Eric de Peyer.)

The technique has potential beyond purely physical improvement and aims to help realize a person's individual potential. It is possible to make the best of whatever situation you find yourself in by the way in which you approach it.

Yoga

We have all heard of the word and perused it from many angles. Some of us get up in the morning and do a few exercises, recite one or two mantras, meditate and then follow our daily lives — we intend to gain something out of the word — peace, tranquillity, love, health, good habits, good rhythm, improved capacity to run, walk, better muscles, younger body and a more effective mind. The first thing we need to know is the meaning of Yoga, its purpose, its function and its aims.

Yoga is an aspect of Hindu philosophy which insists on discipline and acceptance of Theism but its connection to the belief in God is loose. It does not insist on but continuously rises to the thought of God, who is viewed only as a particular soul and no different from any other souls co-existing with Him. His is an eternal connection with the most refined of matter and He is endowed with supreme wisdom and the purest power of goodness.

Aurobindo says: 'Yoga is a double movement of ascent and descent — one rises to higher and higher levels of consciousness, but at the same time one brings down its power, not only to the mind but also in the end, into the body. The highest aim is to achieve the Supermind and to bring that down into all levels of man and the material earth consciousness — this is divine transformation.'

Yoga aims to create a true light in the spirit by controlling and obscuring mental activities. It offers paths which help suppress both the conscious and unconscious activities of the mind, as follows:

MEANS TO ACHIEVE

PRIMARY	Yama and Niyama	Abstention and observance
NECESSITY	Asana and Pranayama	Posture and regulation of breath makes the body yielding and flexible

Pratachara	Withdrawal of the senses from their natural outward functioning provides answers to introversion
Dhyana	Contemplation
Samadhi	Concentration

Yoga, therefore, is not simply confined to calisthenics or breathing exercises but a keen part of the philosophy of understanding and ascending to the finer aspect of Man. It, therefore, has to be taken more seriously than just aiming to get something out of it. It is more a case of enhancing our Being and becoming transcendental. It cannot come out of any mantras, Japas, ceremonies or the like. It is achieved by self adaptation and self absorption of that which is akin to oneself. It must flow with daily living and our *modus operandum*. It must suit the daily living of the king, the soldier, the priest, the tradesman and the various occupational existences. To *adapt* to this, Yoga is divided mainly into four sections.

Hatha Yoga
Aim: A supernormal physical perfection of the body — and through its control, attaining connection with the mental body which in turn attains consciousness of the Divine Being.

This method uses the body and the vital functioning of the body as its instrument for perfection and realization. It is concerned with the gross physical body. All power in the body is stilled, collected, collated, purified, heightened and concentrated to its utmost limits by *Asana* (posture and exercises) and other physical processes such as *Pranayama* (breath absorption). All energy is directed to the physical centre in which Divine Consciousness is concealed in the human body.

It is laborious and makes a very heavy demand on one's time and energy. It demands a complete severance from the ordinary life of men. It is thus very difficult to utilize its results in the daily life of Mankind. One's world becomes void or extraordinarily restricted. On the other hand, it does bring physical results — increased vitality, prolonged youth and vigour, improved health. Is this gain in proportion to the effort?

Raja Yoga
Aims: A supernormal perfection of the capacity of the mental life, which offers a better functioning link with the Divine Being. It aims

to lead from the mere human to the Divine in mankind.

Raja Yoga teaches us to see, know and be divine. It uses the mental being as the power to attain realization. It concentrates on the subtle body. The subtle body is a representation of Soul, amplified by psychic, psychological, mind and brain conditions and processes. It represents the total being. It is that part which is not the body as we see it. The body is a gross form of one's finer being — an extension into material being. By harnessing knowledge, love, mental being, will, heart or intellect, it seeks to arrive at liberating truth.

The ordinary mentality is first disciplined, purified and directed towards the Divine Being. Mind power is developed by concentrated action, achieving supernormal capacities of knowledge, effective will, deep light of perception, powerful light of thought-radiation. It brings one the Yogic or occult powers around which is woven a mystery which is quite dispensible.

Its main instrument (or function) is devotion, which creates powers of the Soul, both emotional and aesthetic. It turns us Godward in perfect Purity and Intensity. This is a *Mental Psychic Process*.

Dharma Yoga
Aims: To raise the human soul to the divine. To use the forces of will, knowledge and love in as pure a form as possible to achieve the purpose of the Divine and with the guidance, example and loving encouragement of a Guru, a master, to achieve the sense of devotion and prayer.

The main instrument is prayer. A prayer is the capacity in one's self to convey and to communicate the deserving part of oneself with a higher Being. It is the capacity to be able to say 'I deserve and therefore be granted'. This promotes effort to deserve and knowledge of what one deserves.

Meditation is also used. This is the capacity to still the mind and live in the presence of an awareness of a thought-free mind. That is, to achieve the liberation and results of absence of thought on the mind and the brain, the brain being the poised instrument of physical action.

Karma Yoga
Aim: To achieve the knowledge of the Self and one's Soul.

This method uses daily living as the lever to control the mind, the body, the mentality, the Psyche and the Divine. The focus remains in the present and the purpose of the present is the Divine Will. One strives to surrender all purpose and action for unity of knowledge, love and will.

In one's everyday life one becomes conscious of the reason for one's birth. The reason being to achieve the knowledge of the Self and one's Soul, but to be purely aware of the unity with all Souls and the Eternal Being.

The four instruments used are:

1. The awareness and knowledge of signs of the truth, the power and the processes that govern realization of the present.
2. Patient, persistent, enthusiastic use of one's personal efforts in the present.
3. Uplifting knowledge and effort into spiritual experience. The direct suggestion, example and influence of a teacher, a Guru, to enable one to live in the present.
4. The use of time — only as a means to measure the cycle of action and a period of divine involvement and not merely for meetings, catching trains and making plans and dating calendars.

In this method, the body, mind, devotion, Hatha Yoga, Raja Yoga, Dharma Yoga are all part of the study of life in the present. Each action, whether it be eating, drinking, walking, seeing, hearing, making love, is for the divine understanding or for better purpose. Awareness and exercising of this awareness is the supreme goal.

Yoga is one of the Six Systems of Indian philosophy. Indian philosophy dates back to 1,500-1,600 BC and its best known period is the epic period 600 BC to AD 200 of which detailed history exists. Buddhism and its offspring, Jainism, brought about a solid revolution in Hindu thinking; it revived the inner core and divided philosophy into six systems, one of them being Yoga. The other five are:

1. Nyaya
This analyses different ways in which knowledge is born, acquired and sustained. Intuition, inference, comparison and verbal testimony are used. To achieve this analysis, one utilizes the five senses — sight, hearing, touch, taste and smell — and one learns to modify the self by better and more precise use of these senses. For the purpose of expression of higher being, one sees and observes; one hears and listens; one touches to feel and think; one tastes food for purity rather than sensual pleasure, one smells the beauty of the finer being.

2. Vaisheshika (Particularly)
This is the study of particular aspects of the world from the Soul — the atom.

3. Sankhya

This system believes in real matter and an infinite variety of individual souls which are not emanations of the single word — *Soul*. A plurality of souls. Cause and effect are the underdeveloped and the developed state of the same substance.

It is a process of liberation by Buddi — intelligence — by a discriminating intelligence. It reflects thoughts by two distinct understandings. 'Vichara' the thought capacity to distinguish right from wrong and 'Vivka' the use of manners and methods of selflessness.

It insists on ascetic renunciation of life and of work as an essential need for liberation. Liberation and renunciation can be seen to be synonymous — true renunciation is the inner rejection of desire and egoism.

4. Purva Mimansa

Dharma. The ascertaining of duty. This system is founded on the belief of the reality of the world and the Individual Souls. It teaches and establishes how every act produces its effect, sometime or other, through the links between the act and the result. The earlier period did not admit to the existence of God, but later teachings do.

5. Vedanta

These are the teachings of the Upanishads and deal with the construction of and the laws governing three worlds, the world of men, the world of elements and the overworld or the world of the gods. These three worlds are joined and the image is used of a cosmic tree, in which the trunk is the world of men, the branches, the world above and the roots the world below. The energies which control the function of the worlds take the form of three 'Gunas', which are defined thus:

Rajas: Positive force; a childlike longing, or blind desire.
Tamas: Negative force; negligence, indolence, sleep.
Satva: A purity, a source of light, a harmonizing force.

The interaction and changing roles of these three principles provide the basis for existence.

Yoga is essentially a part of a complete way of life. Traditionally, a spiritual guide would recommend which path should be given special attention as this obviously varies according to individual needs. Different branches of Yoga are suitable for specific types of people and should not be undertaken without some preparatory self-study and consideration of the needs of one's whole existence.

PART THREE

FIRST AID AND
PATIENT CARE AT HOME

11
THE SICK ROOM

This should be an airy room, especially well ventilated, with an uninterrupted supply of fresh air and a free escape for foul air. The fresh air should come from an open window, but you must make sure that the patient is not in a draught. The ideal temperature for the room should be between 13°C and 16°C (55°F to 60°F) but it can be higher if the patient so desires.

Place the bed so that both sides are easy of access: if possible, there should be a second bed or couch on to which the patient can be moved for a short time each day.

The room should be as quiet as possible, and not contain large quantities of clothing, or anything that might spread infection from one part of the house to another.

A patient suffering from an infectious disease should be separated as far as possible from the rest of the family, and it is best to set aside a room at the top of the house for such cases, since germs, being lighter than air, tend to rise.

The mother or nurse who frequently goes near the patient should know that the illness, though very unwelcome, is only transitory, and keep her courage and morale as high as she humanly can. She should remember that patients, especially children, are likely to feel worse when the nurse is nervous and insecure. Children's pains, in particular, get worse in an atmosphere of insecurity. They become very afraid, which lowers their vitality.

Keep a loose overall near the door and put this on when entering the room. Germs can easily be carried by clothing.

The patient should be sponged over as completely as possible, at least once a day, with water either as warm or as cold as would give comfort. After this he should be quickly and carefully dried with a soft towel. If he finds this exhausting, a small area of the body can be washed at a time until the whole body is completed. It is often thought that if you wash or sponge down a patient who has been sweating badly, he may catch cold, but there is no need for this fear if the sponging is done carefully.

No food should be kept in the sick room, as sometimes the very sight of food can turn the patient against it; also the warmth of the room could make it go bad. He should be tempted to eat by way of surprise, rather than by persuasion.

Flowers should only be kept in the room during the day and removed in the evening when the patient goes to sleep; if left during the night they absorb oxygen.

The patient should be watched and well cared for, but not bothered with a lot of questions; in this way he will be comforted and feel a greater sense of security.

If the patient's temperature is above normal, it is not wise to let him go to the bathroom and take a bath for himself. When he does take his first bath after a spell in bed, there should be someone near to give help, and on no account should he lock the bathroom door.

INVALID DIET

Great care must be taken to ensure that the patient is given the best food. Flagging appetites must be tempted and care must be taken to make food appeal to the eye as well as the palate.

Fresh ripe fruit in season is palatable to an invalid, and can be given in almost all illnesses, even in acute stomach disorders.

In all cases the fruit should be well washed and the skin and pips or seeds removed, whether it is eaten raw or cooked. In the later stages of convalescence the skin should be eaten as normally.

Beverages
Beverages form a major part of an invalid's diet, and great care should be taken that these do not become monotonous. At the beginning of an illness, cold water, soda water, lemon and honey or lemonade, rose-hip syrup, guava juice, grape juice, lemon barley water, blackcurrant juice, apple juice or *Lucozade* are all that are necessary. There is nothing against giving a patient cold or iced water if he so desires, and sucking a small piece of ice can sometimes be helpful.

If the patient becomes tired of sweet and acid drinks and wants something savoury, barley water with a pinch of salt, *Marmite* or *Bovril* may be welcome. Chicken broth and beef tea are very nourishing, but should only be given in small quantities. Teas for everyday use may be found in the tisane section in the Diet chapter.

NOTE: If an invalid diet is prescribed, it is for that patient only, taking into account his individual medical needs, hereditary height-weight ratio, and the remedy he has been given. It will not be suitable for someone else. This also applies to macro and microbiotic, and such other diets which in principle are therapeutic diets, and are not to be adopted as everyday eating habits.

Barley Water. Good for urinary troubles and conditions where a greater formation of urine is required, also extremely useful for digestive disorders. It can be made into a refreshing drink by adding lemon or a little salt.

METHOD: 2 oz barley to 1 pint water. Bring quickly to the boil and let it simmer slowly for half an hour. Strain and cool. Add lemon, glucose or a little salt. The barley removed can be used as one would use rice and need not be thrown away.

Rice Water. Rice water is useful for urinary and digestive troubles. Combined with lemon to provide a vitamin supply; it has a pleasant taste and makes the mouth fresh.

METHOD: 2 tablespoons rice to 1 quart water (prefer brown rice where available). Bring quickly to the boil, and let it simmer for 40 mins. Strain and cool.

Chamomile Tea. Chamomile tea is very useful for toothache, menstrual pains, and nervous tensions; it can be bought at any health food store, or at a chemist. It is supplied either in the form of dried flowers, or else the whole plant is crushed and dried.

METHOD: Put one teaspoon of chamomile tea in a teapot and pour boiling water over it. Allow it to infuse for a few minutes. If you find the taste unpleasant, lemon or honey may be added, or else one teaspoon of chamomile tea to one teaspoon of China tea makes a very pleasant drink.

Hot Lemon
METHOD: 2 teaspoons of lemon juice to an average size tumbler of water. Put the lemon in tepid water, as hot water will disperse the vitamin C.

Hot Lemon and Honey or Glucose
METHOD: Take either a dessertspoon of honey or glucose, and add

a tumbler of hot lemon water prepared as above. A pinch of salt should be added to both if the patient has lost a great deal of fluid by vomiting or diarrhoea.

Beef Tea. This is useful in the second phase of convalescence, when nourishment is needed to build up the patient, and the digestive system is now fully functioning.

METHOD: 1lb fresh beef, ½ teaspoon salt, 1 pint water. Remove all fat and gristle and soak the meat in salty water for half an hour. Bring to the boil in 1 pint fresh water with a little salt, and let it simmer for 3 to 4 hours. The liquid should never be allowed to sink below ½ pint, and should be continually 'topped up' so that there is 1 pint of beef tea at the end.

Semolina
METHOD: 1½ oz semolina to 1 pint of milk. Brown sugar to taste. Mix the semolina into a smooth paste with a little of the milk and bring the rest to the boil, and pour over the mixture, stirring well. Return to the saucepan and let it simmer for 10 to 15 minutes until it thickens. It should then be placed in a dish in a moderate oven for 10 minutes.

Can be served with very small quantity of grated nutmeg, or the juice of a lemon. Very useful early feeding in all those patients who have had gastro-intestinal conditions.

Tapioca. This is made in the same way as a rice pudding in the oven and is used for almost the same reasons. They both form a light convalescent mid-morning feed.

Oatmeal Porridge. This will often help when diarrhoea alternates with constipation. It gives enough vitality and prevents alternate dryness and softness of bowel movements.

Toast. Brown toast is a very good medium for absorbing gastric and bilious disturbances. It is also useful for a hangover. Bread used like this should always be more than three days old; in fact it is always better to eat bread that is at least a day old.

Arrowroot. Arrowroot takes away wind and gas, absorbs foods that are toxic and passes them out the next day in an unconstipated form. It is useful when diarrhoea has set in, and can be taken by adults, children or babies. It is also filling and therefore eases an empty feeling which is often misinterpreted as hunger.

METHOD: 2 teaspoons arrowroot to ½ pint water, or equal parts milk and water. Also equal parts of sour milk or yogurt and water.

Mix the arrowroot into a smooth paste with a little of the cold water or milk, bring the rest to the boil and pour over the mixture, stirring well. Return to the saucepan and simmer slowly for 5 minutes, stirring all the time to stop any lumps from forming. Can be cooked with a little brown sugar but not with white sugar or honey.

12

EMERGENCY TREATMENT

First Aid

First Aid is the help that you can provide until skilled medical aid is available. It is important to yourself, your family and your friends to have a knowledge and understanding of the simple ways in which this can be applied quickly and intelligently. Though you should think in terms of accident prevention, it is vital that in an emergency you have the knowledge and equipment to be of assistance.

You must be observant and tactful, and so learn without thoughtless questions the symptoms and history of the case.

1. Death should never be presumed because signs of life are absent. It is better to treat a dead body than allow a living person to die for want of First Aid.
2. Severe haemorrhage must receive immediate attention even if other injuries are present.
3. If breathing has ceased, artificial respiration must be given. (Method described later.)
4. Patient must be kept warm to arrest fall in temperature and so lessen shock.
5. When the skin is broken the wound should be covered with a clean dressing.
6. When a bone is broken, the patient should not be moved until that bone has been made as immobile as practicable. (Remember *Symphytum* as a remedy.)
7. Poisons swallowed should be emitted by making the patient vomit either mechanically or chemically. If not sure of your action, you would be wise to await expert care.
8. When the patient can swallow, tea may be given as a stimulant, but alcohol should be avoided.

Injuries

The following further points should be observed in dealing with injuries:

1. Germs can very easily be introduced into a wound, so it should be touched as little as possible, and then only with clean hands. If there is a foreign body clearly visible, like glass or metal, this should be removed very gently.
2. A clot of blood should never be disturbed when present over a wound, as it serves the double purpose of keeping blood in and germs out. Always cover a wound with a sterile dressing, kept in place by a bandage.
3. If the wound is dirty, wash it by pouring A.C.U. lotion over it (one teaspoon to a pint of water). If this is not available, use running water; this can be safely considered sterile for all practical purposes of First Aid.
4. When there is serious bleeding, lie the patient down, as blood escapes with less force when a person is sitting or lying. Now raise the bleeding part, but take great care when moving fractures.
5. If bleeding cannot be stopped by bringing the sides of the wound together, or by direct pressure on the wound with fingers or thumb, you may have to apply a tourniquet. In this case call the doctor immediately and remember to tell him about the tourniquet. (If it is covered and he does not know it is there, he may jump to the wrong conclusions.)
6. For bruising and sprains it is best to apply a cold or ice compress. This can be soaked in A.C.U. lotion (teaspoonful to 1 pint of water).

   Indicated remedies include — Arnica, Calendula, Hypericum, Urtica urens.

Object in the throat. Encourage the victim to cough up the object if it cannot be swallowed; on no account probe the throat with your fingers, as this may push the object deeper.

If coughing does not help, get the patient to lean right forward with his head down as far as possible, and slap him hard between the shoulder blades; this should be done very quickly if the object is interfering with the breathing. If the trouble cannot be dislodged, medical aid will be required.

Always see a doctor if the object is not expelled through the mouth, even if the symptoms subside, as any object entering the lungs could cause a cough or infection.

Indicated remedy — Arnica.

Object in the nose. If the object cannot be withdrawn easily or expelled by gentle blowing, you should consult a doctor. Do not probe the nose yourself, or you may push the object deeper and injure the nostril. Do not permit violent nose-blowing.

Swallowed objects. Small round objects like beads, buttons or marbles swallowed by children usually pass uneventfully through the intestines and are eliminated in the normal way. Do not give laxatives or bulky food, just the normal diet, and for several days the stools should be examined to check whether the object has passed. Sharp or straight objects, like hair-pins or open safety pins are dangerous. Consult a doctor, as special instruments and skill are needed to locate such objects.

Dressings and bandages. A dressing is a covering applied to a wound or an injured part. It is usually kept in place by a bandage.

A dry dressing is used to protect a wound. It can be made of lint or gauze and should be sterilized, but in an emergency a perfectly clean handkerchief or piece of linen may be used temporarily.

A wet dressing may be hot or cold. It should be soaked in hot or cold water (or any liquid advised by the doctor) and wrung dry, before being applied to the affected part.

A triangular bandage is the most versatile of bandages. By placing the right-angle point to the centre of the long side, you can quickly fold a broad or narrow bandage as required. Used spread out, it can be turned into a sling, or a covering for the scalp or foot. It can also be used as a splint.

Artificial Respiration

The organs concerned in respiration are: the nose, throat, windpipe (trachea), air tubes (bronchi) and the lungs. As the blood depends upon air for its purification and for oxygen necessary to maintain life, interference with the breathing may very soon cause asphyxia, in drowning, choking, suffocation, etc.

It is best to use the direct method of artificial respiration generally known as the 'Kiss of Life'.

1. Place the patient on his back, and clear mouth and throat of any foreign matter, including dentures.
2. Bring the tongue forward and down, taking care that it does not get bitten; tilt the head back as far as possible, support the chin and maintain this position.

3. Pinch the nostrils to prevent any air from escaping.
4. Take a deep breath and blow into the patient's mouth as though trying to blow up a balloon. Watch for the chest to rise, and if this does not happen, look to see if there is any further obstruction that needs clearing from the throat. Repeat blowing into the mouth every four or five seconds, always moving away in between each blow to allow the breath to escape from the patient's lungs. This should be kept up until normal breathing returns, or a doctor arrives.

It is important to make sure that you yourself do not cause any obstructions to the patient by leaning on the chest, or holding the neck, or even letting your artificial teeth fall into the mouth of the injured.

There is an apparatus available called a 'Brooks Airway', which consists of a plastic tube, a mouth-piece and valve, which is very efficient, and enables the air to go into the lungs without the possibility of the tongue getting in the way. It is also more hygienic.

Acid Burns

These should be washed with water immediately and the patient taken to the doctor.

Burns (Dry and Wet)

Use your common sense with a burn, as in any emergency.

Conventionally, burns are referred to in one of three degrees. In a first degree burn the skin is reddened, in a second degree burn blisters form, and a third degree burn involves destruction of the entire thickness of skin. Body fluid may be easily lost if the burn is bad and threat of shock and infection exists.

Immediate action should be taken to lower the skin temperature. This can be done either by running cold water over the burn until the pain subsides or by wrapping a clean towel that has been immersed in cold water round the affected part.

In the case of a first degree burn apply A.C.U. non-greasy with clean hands and cover with gauze. Clean the next day with A.C.U. lotion. If blisters have formed cover the burn with gauze and do not use ointments as these tend to contain the heat in the burn and prevent the circulation of air to the wound.

Third degree burns should, after cold water treatment, be covered with any clean and ironed teatowel or sheet (if no gauze is available) and taken immediately to hospital. It should be considered as an acute medical condition and not treated at home. A homoeopathic remedy for shock is probably advisable.

A good diet is very important to victims of bad burns. It should be high in protein for tissue repair and plenty of liquids taken. Vitamin C may be helpful for healing the wound and vitamin E may help prevent scarring.

Some indicated remedies — *Arnica.*

Boils
Never squeeze or try to puncture a boil as this may only drive the infection deeper, and delay the recovery. Apply warm, wet compresses soaked in A.C.U. lotion several times a day. When the boil breaks, just wipe away the pus with a pad soaked in the lotion and cover with a sterile dressing.

If you get many boils you should consult your doctor.

Some indicated remedies — *Hepar sulph., Silica.*

Whitlow and Injury to the Nail
Do not try to remove any foreign body from the nail unless you can see it easily. Digging under the nail may damage the skin around it and cause an abscess under the nail — whitlow — which can be extremely painful.

If there is pus and swelling, try placing the finger in hot and ice cold water alternately, and if this does not help, apply a hot kaolin poultice.

It is better to take nail injuries to the doctor unless simple treatment at home succeeds.

Some indicated remedies — *Hepar sulph., Hypericum, Silica.*

Convulsions and Fits
Convulsions are spasmodic and involuntary contractions of the muscles of the body or limbs. In children they are often caused by fever, teething or stomach irritation. If the child becomes rigid with twitching, call the doctor. In the meantime, sit the child for five to ten minutes in a bath of warm water with the knees bent up to the chest, and have a cool sponge ready to apply to the head. Dry the child thoroughly and wrap warmly.

If the bath does not succeed in relieving the child from convulsions, there is no point in repeating it, and it is best to wait until the doctor takes over.

One of the most gruelling experiences is to see a person having an epileptic fit, which is a sudden and complete loss of consciousness, which lasts only a short while. He falls to the ground, sometimes with a scream, and passes into a state of convulsions affecting the whole body. Frothing at the mouth and biting of the tongue may occur.

Treatment. Support the patient's head, and to prevent him biting his tongue, wrap a pencil or something hard in a handkerchief and hold it between his back teeth. Do not forcibly restrain his movements, but wait patiently for the fit to end.

Remedies — With convulsions, treat the cause, e.g. high temperature, etc. With epilepsy, leave it to the doctor after preliminary first aid care.

Cramp in the Night
This is very often a vitamin B deficiency, and even two cramps a month should be reported to the doctor.

A piece of copper can be rubbed on the place where the cramp is. If very severe, a hot water bottle will help.

Some indicated remedies — *Aconite, Cuprium, Mag. phos.* 6 X. Vitamin B_1, about 100mg.

Electric Shock
This is a form of acute shock. The burns are dry and should be treated accordingly.

If the patient is in contact with electricity, it is NOT SAFE to touch him until the current has been turned off at the main. When this is not possible, stout rubber gloves should be used to handle the patient (normal household ones are not thick enough) and if rubber boots are available, put them on. If these things are not at hand, wrap newspaper, rubber or plastic round a broom handle and push the patient away from the current. Make sure everything is absolutely dry, and if the ground is wet, stand on a piece of wood or you may get a shock yourself.

When the patient is away from the current make sure you induce artificial respiration if the breathing has failed.

Some indicated remedies — *Arnica, Calendula, Cantharis, Hamamelis* (Witch Hazel), *Urtica urens.*

Fainting
Place the person on his back, and loosen any tight clothing, especially around the neck and waist. Allow him to get as much fresh air as

possible, and apply a cold compress to his forehead. When he revives, give him hot tea, or if he prefers it, cold water. If the fainting lasts for more than a few minutes, you should get in touch with a doctor.

Fainting may be caused by fatigue, hunger, sudden emotional shock, sight of blood, a poorly ventilated room, etc. The patient's breathing is usually weak, pulse feeble, face pale and the forehead covered with beads of perspiration. Treat the cause wherever possible.

If a person merely feels faint, make him sit in a chair near an open window and bend his forehead between his knees, and tell him to breathe deeply.

Some indicated remedies — *Aconite, Ammon. carb., Ignatia.*

Hiccups
There are several ways of stopping hiccups, but if the attack persists for an hour or more you should consult a doctor.
1. Take a deep breath and hold it for as long as possible.
2. Gargle with plain hot or cold water for a minute or two.
3. Slowly sip several glasses of cold water.
4. Cover your nose and mouth with a paper bag (not on any account plastic); inhale and exhale into it for some minutes.
    The accumulation of carbon dioxide sometimes stops the spasms.

For babies, first try making them belch by patting them on the back. If there is no relief, allow the child to lick a teaspoon which has been dipped in honey, or else moistened and dipped in sugar.

Some indicated remedies — *Aconite, Arnica, Ignatia.*

Nose Bleeds
Repeated nose bleeding is a medical problem, but it is important to know how to tackle an individual nose bleed. Try to make sure that no blood is swallowed, and it is best to sit the patient down and drop his head forward. If he is inclined to faint, put his head between his knees and apply a cold compress to his head. If he is not feeling faint, put his head under a cold tap. Loosen clothes and anything tight round the neck, and give him as much fresh air as possible.

Never lie a patient on his back and do not let him blow his nose.

Shock
Shock is a condition of sudden depression of the nervous system, and can be expected after any serious injury or sudden illness. It may vary from a slight feeling of faintness to a condition of collapse

in which the vital forces of the body are exhausted.

The skin is pale, cold and clammy; the pulse rapid, breathing shallow, rapid or irregular; the injured person is frightened, restless and often apprehensive.

Keep him lying down, and loosen his clothing; keep him well covered but do not cause sweating. If he is thirsty, give him a little plain cold water, a few sips at a time. Never give alcohol or stimulants.

Remember, shock will be increased by: loss of blood; exposure to cold; severe pain; mental anxiety; and these factors should be alleviated as soon as possible.

Some indicated remedies — *Aconite, Arnica, Carbo veg., Ignatia, Natrum sulph., Rhus tox., Urtica urens.*

Stings and Bites

Apply cold fomentation with vinegar, one teaspoon to a pint of water. Always, if possible, remove the sting with a pair of tweezers. Local applications of *Apis* 3 liquid is extremely helpful. Dilute A.C.U. liquid will often serve the same purpose.

Extreme allergies to insect bites need a doctor's attention.

Sudden severe swelling of the whole body is well relieved by *Aconite*, or by use of *Apis* 3, 10 drops taken every few minutes until the swelling subsides.

Sunburn

Every year we have many severe cases of sunburn caused by physical 'worship of the sun', rather than the spiritual form as in India. When the damage is severe, there may be other effects such as headaches, vomiting, diarrhoea and dysentry.

You should never sun-bathe for more than twenty minutes without going into the shade, particularly in the middle of the day. The ultra-violet rays are most beneficial during the first few minutes of sunrise and before sunset, so sun-bathing should be done at these times if practicable!

Sunflower oil or any bland oil may be applied to the skin before it is exposed to the sun, and A.C.U. ointment may be used freely if there is any soreness. Ordinary sun-lotions, some of which colour the skin, are harmful, especially those you get abroad (because in many countries there is no restriction on the use of cortisone in lotions).

Sunstroke is a severe and drastic illness caused by over-exposure to the sun; it is only sunburn, but to a more severe degree. It needs immediate medical care.

Some indicated remedies — *Arnica, Belladonna, Ferrum phosphoricum, Hypericum, Natrum sulph., Urtica urens.*

Travel Sickness

This should be considered as an acute condition, and the person's reactions as a whole should be studied. If this is a condition which occurs regularly, even on short journeys and under normal conditions, the doctor should be consulted. Drugs should not be taken for travel sickness, as when these are used the patient will take time to accommodate himself after the journey. If there is fear of a journey, and some travel sickness is caused by the anxiety in undertaking a journey in case one is sick — *Arg. nit* or *Gelsemium* may be considered.

Homoeopathic remedies should preferably be used only in bad cases and during long journeys.

Arg. nit. See Remedy (Feeling of being shut in and anticipation.)

Gelsemium. See Remedy (Anxiety about future event.)

Pulsatilla. See Remedy (Cabin sickness. Wants fresh air.)

Tobaccum. Nausea, giddiness, vomiting, icy coldness and sweat. Extreme prostration. Feels terribly faint. Faint sick feeling in pit of stomach. Sickness caused by petrol, diesel and engine fumes. Vomits at least motion. Vomiting of pregnant women who are not otherwise subject to travel sickness. Better in fresh air.

Cocculus. Sickness, especially car sickness caused by looking at moving objects, or seeing the sea from a rocking boat. Worse on becoming cold. Better for avoiding seeing motion.

Baptisia. Sickness due to smell of food, unable to eat or drink anything that has a smell. Cannot enter a dining room when travelling.

Petroleum. Sickness is caused through sensations in the ears, throbbing of engines, boat and aeroplane engines. Sickness is accompanied by feeling of emptiness in stomach, although the person has eaten. Eating gives very little or no comfort to the 'empty, gone' nausea sensation. Better in warm air and lying with head high.

13

SOME COMMON AILMENTS

Colds and Coughs

The term 'cold' is such a misnomer that it cannot be defined. However, the common cold is common knowledge.

Colds are often caused by draughts of cold air, shoes that let the water in, or wet boots and clothes. Wet feet and damp clothes do not necessarily result in a cold so long as you change into warm dry things as soon as possible. It is not when you are hot that you are susceptible to a cold, but when you are cooling down: a cold may be produced by getting chilled after sweating, or from insufficient clothing when the body is hot after exercise. Make sure you have enough clothing.

Remember also that damp beds, prolonged bathing, passing from heated areas into cold ones, and insufficient rest after an illness, are very common causes of colds.

There are certain types of colds that should not be treated with a remedy: for instance, if the body as a whole is not involved but only the nose and throat, it is a sign that something in the respiratory tract needs to be thrown away. Colds that give a thick, pus-like smelly discharge are very often part of this eliminative process. The first cold in a change of season or weather comes into this category: it is throwing out the old immunity forces and creating new ones; new antibodies are being produced against new organisms with which you have not yet learnt to live, and these antibodies help to build up the body's resistance to different diseases. If you try to suppress this cold you may suffer from many more during the season, so it is important to let your body become acclimatized as best you can.

These colds can be overcome with hot lemon and honey drinks, hot water gargles, rest and warmth, good breathing and plenty of fresh air. The whole thing should clear up after a little sneezing and discomfort.

It is important to increase your supply of vitamin C; one way is by ascorbic acid tablets. Normal dosage for an adult must never exceed 1g divided doses per day, and children 0.5g in divided doses per day. On the second and third days the doses should be reduced by half each day. (Don't take them indefinitely or they will actually lead to a cold.) Better still, take plenty of fresh lemon, honey and fruit juice. I have seen people get over colds in a matter of hours by sipping luke-warm lemon juice with honey well dissolved in it. Never add boiling water to fruit juice or much of the value of the vitamins is lost.

In all such colds the ideal treatment is rest, uniform warmth, hot hip or foot-baths, warm light food with sparing use of meat and eggs, but plenty of sour milk, honey and lemon. The main need is good hygiene, common sense eating, fresh air, warmth and rest.

The treatment of chronic colds should be left to the physician.

Some indicated remedies — *Aconite, Allium cepa, Arsenicum album, Belladonna, Bryonia, Carbo veg., Kali bic., Kali carb., Pyrogenium, Pulsatilla, Rhus tox.*

Coughs
Some indicated remedies — *Aconite, Allium cepa, Bryonia, Calendula, Carbo veg., Chamomilla, Hepar sulph., Kali bic., Kali carb., Mercurius, Nux vomica, Rhus tox., Ruta, Silica.*

Diabetes
Diabetes is a metabolic disorder, characterized by decreased ability, or complete inability, of the body to utilize carbohydrates. Therefore there is an insufficiency or absence of insulin. At this point insulin is usually over-prescribed which results in the disuse atrophy of the islets of Langerhans, which is that part of the pancreas which produces insulin. My personal approach is to put the patient on a diet to reduce the need for insulin or to combine the diet with glucophages — orally administered insulin supplements — in order to balance the blood sugar.

Only as a last resort should insulin be injected and then a quantity that demands the maximum use of the islets of Langerhans. The homoeopath uses the *remedia constitutionalis* to stimulate the pancreas and above all, refuses to recognize the incurability of the disease.

It should be noted that insulins are often combined with zinc or cobalt in order to prolong their effective life within the body. Over a prolonged period these substances may cause side-effects and a remedy may have to be chosen for this condition.

Diarrhoea

As in all illnesses, every case of diarrhoea has a cause, and it is that cause we ought to treat. The number of stools are of less consequence than the general health of the patient. It is important not to suppress diarrhoea, or else it will be followed by constipation and a return of diarrhoea. Diarrhoea is the repeated formation of a liquid stool (not one large liquid stool). It is often part of an eliminative process, and can be treated without a special homoeopathic remedy: for instance, by going without usual food, and taking plenty of liquids, especially with salts and minerals, to replace what the body has lost. If you do not replace these, serious illnesses may follow. The aim, therefore, is to form a more healthy stool and not only to stop unhealthy frequency.

In a child, where the intestines are not so well formed and matured, anatomically, as in an adult, diarrhoea and vomiting can occur more easily. Fluid and mineral losses take place very quickly, making the child dehydrated. (Remember, too, that thin people become dehydrated more easily than fat people.) Make sure that enough liquids are taken, like glucose water (1 tablespoon to a pint of water), rice water, or barley water, thus replacing body fluids and minerals.

Arrowroot, oatmeal porridge, tapioca and semolina are all useful foods for a disturbed digestive system, as they absorb a great deal of toxic material from the bowels. These foods have an invigorating influence in themselves, but if the patient is feeling extremely weak, glucose may be added.

In a bout of diarrhoea, the temperature should be taken frequently. Severe diarrhoea is often accompanied by fever. If the temperature is high you should consult the doctor, as the digestive disturbance is due to an infection and therefore to be diagnosed, understood and treated.

Fever

Fever should not be regarded as an enemy; it is a condition of the body in which there is a rise of temperature that can be registered by a thermometer. Always remember that a fever is an index of a bodily process whereby in raising the temperature the body is reacting to conditions within itself. These conditions may be due to external causes such as getting chilled inside through being cold, or being out in a storm and not changing wet clothes, or even just getting wet feet. On the other hand, it may be an indication that the body is fighting an infection, and is physiologically needing the temperature to aid its cure. There are rare conditions in the body where temperature may rise as a result of a thermal centre disturbance, but we need not go into that here.

Before consulting the doctor about a rise in temperature you should think of it not in terms of a major disturbance that must at all costs be resolved by adopting methods to reduce it, but as an indication that the body is needing help and rest. It is necessary, therefore, to go to bed, be warm and well wrapped up, and give the body generally the help it is asking for.

Unless the temperature is very high, wait and see if the body will cope with the situation in its own way. If it is unable to do so, then consider a remedy, but treat the fever as only one symptom and not the main problem. As in all conditions of the body, study the patient as a whole before choosing the remedy.

Headaches

Repeated and continuous headaches are a doctor's problem, which you should not treat for yourself but bring to his notice.

For the occasional severe headache there are several remedies which will help, but first it is necessary to discover the cause and identify the type of pain.

One of the main causes of headaches is over-indulgence: over-eating, eating wrong things or food that particularly does not suit you, or drinking too much alcohol. Other causes could be mental or physical fatigue, working under pressure, anxiety, emotional strain, mental or sexual frustration, reading too late at night, menstruation or the start of a cold or influenza.

In the case of eating too much or eating the wrong thing, the best cure is to give the stomach a rest for a while so that some of the excess food can be digested. A walk in the fresh air or some form of exercise may be helpful.

Alcoholic Headache

If possible, get rid of the alcohol by vomiting. This can be achieved by active physical irritation such as a finger, a piece of string or a feather against the back of the throat. It may also be induced by chamomile tea or hot lemon water with a pinch of mustard. As you will have already absorbed a good deal of alcohol into the system, it is advisable either to sweat it out of the body, or to urinate more. Lemon and barley water will help this. Excessive alcohol upsets the liver and causes a great deal of congestion, the bile does not circulate properly, and this produces a disturbance. There is no remedy that can be taken in anticipation of a hangover, and if you have too many hangovers the liver will suffer, so spare it as much as you can. If you have been drinking spirits, a small quantity of beer may help to clear the head and vice versa; if the cause is too much wine, then a small quantity of wine in a large glass of soda water may help.

Some headaches are relieved by placing a cold compress of cider vinegar on the forehead. This can be prepared by taking a cup of ice-cold water and adding a dessertspoon of cider vinegar.

Headaches due to an on-coming cold are best treated with some form of vitamin C, such as ascorbic acid, say a 500mg tablet, dissolved in a large glass of water. This should not be repeated more than once. Plenty of fresh orange and lemon juice will help, also lemon and honey in warm water.

Headaches due to menstruation should be treated as you would a menstrual pain.

Some indicated remedies — *Aconite, Arnica, Belladonna, Carbo veg., Chamomilla, Chelidonium, Gelsemium, Nux vomica, Staphysagria.*

Indigestion and Constipation

Indigestion is one of the most common complaints that the physician has to treat. The symptoms vary greatly both in character and in intensity, but there is usually one or more of the following: impaired appetite, flatulence, nausea and eructations which often bring up bitter or acid fluids, furred tongue, foul taste or breath, heartburn, pain, sensation of weight, feeling of fullness after a meal, irregular action of bowels, headache and diminished mental energy and alertness.

Indigestion is often caused by irregularities in diet, too much rich or highly seasoned food, eating too quickly or too frequently, imperfect mastication; or on the other hand by going without food for too long. The digestive system is also the first to suffer from depression and anxiety. When the mind is depressed by disappointment or worry, there is a corresponding depression of the nerve energies; so the stomach, in common with other organs, loses vital energy.

When there is discomfort, you must ask yourself whether it is possible either to pass wind above or below, and if any relief is obtained from this. If you wish to pass wind below and cannot do so, a charcoal biscuit is often helpful. You may also use a glycerine suppository.

If the cause of the pain is something that you have been eating or drinking, then the best answer is to take a pinch of mustard in a glass of hot water and be sick, so letting out the cause of the pain. If you do this, you should also have some warm lemon and honey afterwards to soothe the stomach.

Constipation
Constipation means different things to different people. It should be considered a medical problem if you suffer from it constantly. It is a frequent problem with young children and babies, and can be caused by a change of diet or conditions, which precipitates either a bloated abdomen or an ineffective urge to pass a stool.

The main treatment is dietetic: providing plenty of fruit roughage and fluids should cure the trouble.

However, in an acutely uncomfortable condition the best treatment is a glycerine suppository. Gently lubricate the rectum with A.C.U. ointment or oil, and insert the adult size (infant size is only for children under five years). Encourage the patient to hold the suppository in the rectum for twenty minutes, but a definite urge need not be held back.

Use of mild laxatives, like charcoal biscuits, cascara, senna pods or sennacots can be permitted, provided one is absolutely certain that the cause of constipation is change of habitat, diet, country, etc.

If there is pain in the abdomen accompanied by vomiting and diarrhoea, it is important that no purgatives of any kind should be given without a doctor's instructions. A wandering pain around the umbilicus may gradually settle on the right side of the abdomen with a slight fever, and could be an indication of appendicitis, in which case a purgative is most dangerous.

Some indicated remedies — *Ars. alb., Bryonia, Carbo veg., Discorea, Nux vomica, Pulsatilla.*

Influenza
Influenza is a virus infection, carried through the bloodstream and so through the body as a whole. There is usually a fever, and at advanced stages (but only then) there will be shivers of the inner organs, with anxiety and fear of death. Influenza very often occurs in epidemics, and the remedy epidemicus will have been found within a few days; so ring your doctor, if you have influenza and there are many cases around you, for the name of the remedy epidemicus.

There are various preventive methods and vaccines suggested by homoeopathic chemists and patients; most of these are plausible but not necessarily satisfactory. However, in my experience, if a proper remedy is chosen quickly and the patient has good and immediate rest and reasonably sensible diet, he will recover in a short while.

Some indicated remedies — *Aconite, Arsenicum album, Bryonia, Eupatorium, Gelsemium, Nux vomica, Pyrogenium, Rhus tox.*

Post-Influenzal Depression
Treatment for this is very important, and an episode in itself because influenza leaves you highly depressed.

Some indicated remedies — *Kali phos., Pulsatilla.*

Menstrual Pain
Pain must have a cause, and if you have this type of pain you will probably have discussed it with your doctor during a consultation. Relief may be obtained from 'common-sense' treatment, like more rest, a hot water bottle or a hot drink. If this does not help, a remedy can be considered; but do not just take a remedy and not rest. Also avoid severe strain and strenuous exercise.

Some indicated remedies — *Arsen. alb., Carbo veg., Chamomilla, Kali phos., Mag. phos.*

Piles
Most cases of painful piles can be relieved by the use of hot and cold compresses, and A.C.U. ointment is the ideal lubricant to bring acute relief. A bidet is an invaluable aid in the home, as an alternate spray of hot and cold water can be administered easily.

Acute haemorrhoids are very often associated with sitting on cold floors, or a hard seat, long travels, constipation, and after childbirth. Drinking buckwheat tea for a while may be helpful for this condition. If a remedy is indicated, it should be chosen with the help of your doctor.

Some indicated remedies — *Aconite, Aesculus, Calc. phos., Carbo veg., Hamamelis, Ratanhia* (excruciating pain).

Rheumatism
This is a subject in itself. The word has many meanings, from the simplest aches and pains to extreme rheumatic complaints in muscles and bones. The main theme, however, relates to the muscles, joints, and bones of the locomotor system. Rheumatism is a chronic condition which will need medical care, but you can take various

steps yourself to alleviate minor aches and pains.

Muscles are extremely sensitive to heat, damp, cold, humidity and atmospheric electricity. They are also sensitive to proper and improper use of the body and to the right or wrong blood supply. In most cases, this susceptibility also has a good or bad effect on the joints and bones. Thus, except for rheumatic conditions caused by trauma (injury) involving joints and bones, most rheumatism is blood-borne, due to bad use of the body, bad blood supply, or strong external influences, such as changes in the weather, damp beds, etc.

The proper use of the muscles and the correct carriage of the body can help to eliminate many serious disorders. There are various ways of teaching this, including the Alexander Technique and Yoga methods.

In the case of blood-borne conditions, homoeopathic care is also needed. Homoeopathy is also most helpful when the body is extremely sensitive to external influences.

It is when the blood stream carries toxic materials, owing to bad diet or illness, or over-all carelessness in the use of the body, that the aches and pains begin in the muscles. If you treat these aches and pains with aspirin, codeine, cortisone and such drugs, a general body failure will soon follow. Acid and crystalline deposits will form in the muscles and joints, and then in the bones, resulting in severe and lasting pains and deformities.

The main theme of rheumatism is that when pain begins, there is a tendency to tense and get stiff in areas above and below. For example, if the elbow is painful, the wrist and shoulder stiffen and tense, thus lessening the blood supply to the aching part and so causing congestion, disease and more pain. So remember, while it is important to rest and immobilize a painful joint, it is equally important to keep the parts above and below the painful area fully mobile. If in this way you rest the painful parts and use the pain-free parts properly, you will stop a vicious circle setting in, which will mean losing more and more movement.

Such practices as wearing copper bracelets have a scientific basis. Copper is a trace mineral in the body and meant to give electrical stability. When you wear copper, traces are absorbed and the rest of it helps to render harmless any external electrical influences. When you wear these bracelets, remember that the body has polarity, and the copper should be worn on the negative side. In a right-handed person, the right side of the body is positive and the left negative; the other way round in a left-handed person.

Diet plays an important part. Acid-forming foods like meat, milk and eggs should be avoided, as should rhubarb, spinach, strawberries and tomatoes. Fatty foods also tend to cause increased acids.

Rheumatic people can benefit from a vegetarian diet, but only if the balance of protein, carbohydrate and fat is properly maintained. The Western vegetarian tends to neglect his protein intake and eats too much carbohydrates and fats: too many nuts and too much cheese, for instance. Both these foods are rich in fat and difficult to digest. In the East, this protein imbalance is corrected by whey (sour milk from which the fat has been removed) or by lentils. There are many varieties of lentils, but few of these are known or used in the West; any Eastern cookery book* will solve this problem, and also show what great reliance is placed in the East on raw foods and vegetables.

Sleeplessness

This is often caused by nervous tension such as worry, anxiety, mental activity, or excitement, or else by digestive conditions. It may be due to shock, or being over-tired mentally or physically, and it is important to know the cause before choosing a remedy.

Avoid stimulants such as alcohol or coffee in the evening. The occasional use of Linden tea may be helpful.

Some indicated remedies — *Aconite, Arsenicum album, Arnica, Carbo veg., Chamomilla.*

Cina — sudden distressing crisis in a child with worms — needs to be rocked to sleep violently.

Coffea — excessive mental and physical excitement.

Cocculus — thinks of business, an actor of his act, fatigue of night watchman.

Gelsemium — languid, but cannot compose mind.

Ignatia, Kali. bic., Natrum mur., Nux vomica, Pulsatilla, Rhus tox.

Sticta — after operations and teeth extractions.

Staphysagria.

* *For instance: Eastern Vegetarian Cooking* by Madhur Jaffrey (Cape). Available in the USA as *World of the East Vegetarian Cooking* (Knopf, N.Y.).

PART FOUR

CATALOGUE OF REMEDIES

INTRODUCTION

This section of the book presents the symptom picture of some forty remedies. These symptom pictures are all based on the original remedy provings made by Hahnemann. You may find their wording a little strange; they are presented thus partly because Hahnemann wished his words retained and also because experience constantly reiterates the precision of his findings.

Unless you have carefully read and studied the first sections of this book you will find this section of no practical use. If you read through the symptom pictures and choose the first remedy that seems to fit your symptoms, it will almost certainly be less effective than one chosen after adequate study of homoeopathic principles.

A badly chosen remedy can cause difficulties for the physician, as the incorrect remedy will create a new set of symptoms in the patient, overlaid on the symptoms of the illness. Also, if the remedy is incorrect, the pathological process of the illness will continue unhindered and, in certain cases, the remedy will directly cause the pathology of the illness to change. (For example: if one mistakenly took *Hepar sulph.*, to help heal an abscess, when one should have taken *Silica*, the abscess will suppurate and not resolve itself.) Remedies are inter-related; some contradict each other and are not compatible; others are complementary and help to perpetuate the action of different remedies that may have been taken beforehand. Obviously, remedies must be chosen with great care. Get to know them gradually.

It is very important that you should know when to choose a remedy and when to leave it to the doctor. What are the alternatives? Can the condition be relieved by common-sense treatment such as a change of diet or a period of rest? If the condition is chronic you must call the doctor. If you have decided to choose a remedy, have you made a careful note of all the patient's symptoms before turning to this section of the book to study the remedy pictures? There are no short cuts to the correct decision. You must first have an understanding of the principles of homoeopathy and then follow a systematic and orderly means of application such as I have laid out in the first section of the book.

In the following catalogue of remedies I have arranged Hahnemann's findings in an order that corresponds to basic homoeopathic principles; in particular, the principle of recovery as described in the paragraph on 'Symptoms and Recovery'. You may also note that several of the remedies are not included in the Home Chest, especially under the headings 'Compare' (for similar remedies) and 'Antidote' (for directly opposite ones), which counteract certain other remedies. There is also a heading 'Complementary' which refers to those remedies which help each other. This is to enable those interested in studying homoeopathy further to proceed to a more advanced stage.

REMEDIES

Before reading this section, please read again Chapter One and especially pages 24-25. I emphasize that the 'Characteristics' given for a remedy are its 'provings'.

Aconite (Monkshood)
Useful remedy in the beginning of an acute illness, but must not be continued after a pathological change takes place. Its action is brief and is normally indicated only within the first 24 hours. Strong and healthy people get into this condition through sudden changes of climate, or exposure to cold winds. Patient may have rapid bouncing pulse. Tension in body and blood vessels. Great fear and anxiety. Restless and tossing about. Pains are intolerable. The condition is sudden. Severe. Acute anxiety. Wakes in the middle of the night feeling sure he is going to die.

Sleeplessness. Restless, excited, tossing, full of anguish. Fear of death. Sudden chill. Useful in any condition that comes on suddenly in the night when *Aconite* will give peace and sleep. Useful for insomnia in the aged.

Headache. Very typical headache, can scarcely be described. Comes on with sudden violence. Tearing, burning pain in scalp. Fullness and heaviness of the forehead. Feels as if contents of brain will be forced out. Mild headache with restlessness. Anguish, fever, fear. Worse from cold winds.

Colds and Sore Throat. Cold is sudden. Dry nose. Severe headache. Fluent running nose with much sneezing. Throat is inflamed. Very red tingling throat. Feeling of acute inflammation. Difficult to swallow. Burning, smarting dryness. Larynx is sensitive. May have high temperature.

Coughs. Cough comes on suddenly. Constant short dry cough. Wakes him from his sleep. Worse from loud speaking. Worse after exposure to cold dry winds. No expectoration, except perhaps a little watery mucus or blood. A child has an agonizing cough. Tightness of chest, but not much wheezing. Tosses about, restless, with short dry cough.

Earache. Acute pain. Very sensitive to noises, music is unbearable. External ear hot, red and swollen. Condition comes on suddenly.

Influenza (Breakbone fever). Sudden onset of fever with chilliness. Throbbing pulse. Great restlessness. Anxiety. Thirst and restlessness always present. Cold sweat and icy coldness of face. Chilly if uncovered or touched. Cold waves pass through him. Alternate coldness and heat. Symptoms relieved by sweating. Evening chilliness soon after going to bed.

Measles. High fever. Catarrh. Redness of eyes. Congestion. Barking cough. Itching burning skin. Restlessness and tossing about. Anxiety. Fear. You usually find the patient has been in contact with measles.

Eyes. Foreign bodies in the eyes can often be removed by using *Aconite* 200 — a single dose only.

Piles. Useful remedy for bleeding haemorrhoids, with pain and nightly itching and stitching in anus.
Better — in open air. After sweating. Rest.
Worse — in a warm room, in the evening and at night, lying on left and on affected side, from music, tobacco smoke, dry cold winds and motion.
Complementary: *Coffea, Sulph.*

Allium cepa (Red Onion)
Characteristics: Picture of acrid coryza and bland eye discharge. Think of the appearance of a person who has been cutting up onions. Burning in nose, throat, bladder and skin. Sensation of glowing heat on different parts of the body.

Eyes. Bland discharge, leaving no ulceration or redness afterwards. Burning and smarting, sensitive to light. Conjunctivitis. Hay fever.

Colds and Coughs. Coryza, fluent, acrid, burning nasal discharge, with burning in larynx. A singer's cold. Hay fever. Hoarseness with hacking cough. Tickling in larynx, as if it were torn and split. Pain extending to the ear.

Worse — In the evening. In a warm room.
Better — Open air. In a cold room.
Compare: *Gelsemium, Eupatorium, Aconite, Ipecac.*
Complementary: *Phos., Thuja., Puls.*
Antidotes: *Arnica, Chamomilla, Baryta carb.*

Apis mellifica (Honey Bee)

Characteristics: Like a bee. Fussy, fidgety, jealous, sharp, screaming, suspicious and swollen. Restless, anxious, confused, awkward. Sinks into unconsciousness rather rapidly. Symptoms appear fr m right to left. Thirstlessness. Bluish, pale puffiness that puts on pressure. Localized inflammation, oedematous swellings. People allergic to penicillin.

Eyes. A great remedy for the eyes. Stinging and stitching pains bette for cold, and cold bathing. Cannot stand heat of fire. Extreme oedema. Swelling of the rim of eyelids which may be enormous, looking like raw beef. Profuse weeping. Inability to bear light.

Throat. Oedema of the uvula.

Chest. Dyspnoea due to oedema of lungs.

Rectum. Diarrhoea with a feeling of an open anus.

Urinary. Suppression of urine. Casts in urine. Acute and chronic nephritis.

Skin. Swellings after bites of insects. Sore, sensitive, stinging.

NOTE: In oedemas give lower potencies. Low potencies should not be given in pregnancy. The remedy is slow-acting.
Worse — From 3-5 p.m. After sleep. In a closed room. All forms of heat, hot application, warm drinks. Touch. Pressure. Right side.
Better — In open air. Uncovering. Cold bathing.
Compare: *Apium virus, Cantharis, Lachesis, Vespa, Zinc.*
Complementary: *Nat. mur., Baryta carb.*, if lymphatics involved.
Inimical: *Rhus.*

Argentum nitricum (Nitrate of silver)
A most important remedy yet one that should be selected with care.

Characteristics: Prize neurotic. Master rationalizer. King of liars and belchers. Fearful and nervous. Hurried, worried and scared, impulsive, wants to do everything in a hurry. Feeling that someone is following him in the street. He must walk fast. Suffers from claustrophobia. Lacks confidence. Stage fright of actors. (Remember stage fright is *Argent. nit.* while stage nerves is *Gelsemium.*) Afraid of crowds, heights and failure, rather than death. Melancholic. Complaints due to anticipation. Difficulty in sleeping, with visions of dead at night. Sexy dreams. Makes mountains out of molehills.

Headache. Headache with coldness and trembling. Pain from mental exertion or dancing. Sense of expansion. Boring pain, better on tight bandaging and pressure. Headache better in cold. Headache from stimulants. Vertigo.

Sore throats. Raw, rough and sore. Hoarseness as of cinders. Sensation as if a splinter in the throat. Thick mucus in the throat which causes coughing. Hoarseness is for high sounds rather than low ones.

Stomach. Stomach troubles are accompanied by belching, very difficult and explosive, after which the patient feels better. Belching after meals. Painful feeling in pit of stomach. Feeling as if stomach would burst. Craving for sugar and sweets which do not agree with him. Desire for cheese and salt. Red painful tip of tongue. Travel sickness caused by height rather than motion or rolling rocking movements.

Diarrhoea. Offensive. Instantly after eating or drinking, as though everything goes straight through. Green stools like chopped spinach.

Menstruation. Early. Profuse, long-lasting. Fainting with menses. Pain in uterus during menses. Haemorrhage after intercourse in people otherwise healthy.

Worse — In summer. At night. After eating. From cold food and sweets. Warmth in any form. Left side. During stools. Excitement. Anticipation.

Better — In cold weather. Fresh air. Cold. Pressure. Pain in the back is better standing up.

Compare: *Ars. alb., Merc., Phos., Pulsatilla.*
Antidotes: *Nat. mur.* Therefore cannot be used before or after it.

NOTE: When taking *Argent. nit.* the patient should be taken off salt.

Arnica (Leopard's Bane)
Master remedy for shock.

Characteristics: Patient is bruised, sore, tender, and resents being touched. Bed feels too hard, sensation of falling from bed. Limbs and body ache as if beaten. Stupor, but answers correctly when roused. Useful remedy for sprains, concussion, and after-effects of blows or falls. For painful eruptions and bedsores, remember *Arnica* (A.C.U. ointment). Nervous, cannot bear pain, whole body oversensitive. Useful remedy after mental strain or shock.

Sleeplessness. Too tired to sleep. Bed feels too hard. Body feels sore and tender. Restless when over-tired. Must move to try for relief. Useful remedy for sleeplessness after exertion, physical injuries or mental strain.

Shock. While answering question patient falls into deep stupor before finishing. Useful remedy for mechanical injuries. Bruises, sprains, concussion and their after-effects. Depressed vitality from shock. Shock from mental or physical cause. Patient cold with pallor and drowsiness.

Earache. Caused by local injuries, blast of air or sand, height pressures. Humidity. Pain in the outer ear due to frost-bite, colds, draughts and local injuries. Water in the ear after diving.

Toothache. Useful remedy that can be taken before a visit to the dentist, and while undergoing dental treatment. For pain after extraction of tooth, and after painful fillings, especially when bruised during dental procedures; where a nerve has been exposed and treated, it can be alternated with *Hypericum* (same potency).

Headache. Aching pain in the temples. Burning in head and brain. Rest of body is cool. Great shoots of pain when coughing or sneezing. Cutting in head as if from a knife. Great coldness in body. Bed feels hard. Ordinary pillow too hard for head. Confused.

Pains. All pains anywhere, rheumatism, or any condition where 'as if bruised all over' is a major symptom.

Burns. Useful remedy for shock and pain from burns. *Arnica* (A.C.U. ointment) can be applied to burns as directed on page 111.

Menstrual Pains. Alternate with mental depression. Pains as if kicked and bruised in the lower abdomen.

Worse — Least touch, motion, rest, wine, damp cold, beginning to lie down.

Better — Lying down or with head low.
Antidotes: *Camphor.*
Complementary: *Aconite.*
Compare: *Aconite, Rhus tox., Hypericum, Baptisia.*

Arnica, Calendula and Urtica urens (A.C.U. lotion and ointment)
These have been discussed as separate remedies and they combine
in equal quantities to form a most useful lotion and 2% ointment
which can be used for many purposes in the home.

Lotion. Can be used for washing all burns, cuts, bruises, contusions,
lacerations and wounds, two teaspoons to a pint of water. It should
be used 1:4 for dressing purposes.

There is no need for a dressing when the outer surface of the skin
is not broken, but it is advisable to use the ointment.

Ointment. This is most useful for bruises, grazes, sore and chapped
skin, and can be applied to burns of all kinds, including sunburn.
It may be used quite safely on septic spots or sores. It can also be
used for an injury that has practically healed up, when no further
dressing is needed, and the wound can be kept exposed.

It is a multi-purpose ointment, and can be obtained in a greasy
and non-greasy form, non-greasy being used for absorbent surfaces
and where cosmetic necessity would prevent use of grease, e.g. on
face. One family, which calls it Cuts, Burns, Bruises ointment, has
christened it C.B.B.

Arnica, Calendula and *Urtica* can be bought as mother tinctures
or fluid extracts. Mother tinctures, which are the basis of
homoeopathic remedy making, are very costly; and fluid extracts,
which are much less expensive, are quite satisfactory.

Arsenicum album (Arsenious Acid)
Patient, in spite of illness, is constantly worried about tidiness.
Fastidious. Intolerant of disorderly smells, or disorder around him.
Anxious, restless, afraid of being left alone, afraid of death. Is
suspicious of his medicine. Loves to think of money. Patient faint,
prostate, lacks vitality. Chilly. Burning pains which are better for
heat, except headaches which are better for cold application. Thirst
for cold water, taken frequently in small sips, and is worse for it. Great
exhaustion after slightest exertion. Very ancient remedy, men once
used it to enable them to run long distances. Also used for improving
horses' skin. In acute cases it is very seldom the remedy that effects

the complete cure, a further remedy will be needed six to eight hours later, or the patient may become very disturbed. Mainly right-sided. Predominantly useful for vegetarians.

Headache. Burning pains with restlessness. Cold skin. Sensitive head in open air. Scalp is so sensitive that he cannot brush his hair. Although patient is better from heat, his headaches are worse for it.

Vomiting and Diarrhoea. Burning pain in abdomen, relieved by heat. Cannot bear the sight or smell of food. Great thirst, but drinks little at a time. Vomiting of grass-green solids or fluids. Nausea, retching and vomiting after eating and drinking. Distended and painful abdomen. Sensitive to slightest touch. Anxious about his stomach. Rice-water stools with blood but very little mucus. Diarrhoea and vomiting worse between 1 a.m. and 3 a.m. Better for small sips of hot tea or water. Useful remedy for ill effects of vegetable diet, melons and watery fruits — diarrhoea alternating with constipation.

Haemorrhoids or Piles. Patient has sudden acute piles, with stitching pain when walking and sitting, but not at stool. Pain in piles is better when passing a stool. Burning pains around the anus, relieved by hot water. Tenesmus, rectal pain with spasmodic reaction.

Menstruation. Pain as from red-hot wires. Worse least exertion, which causes great fatigue. Stitching pain in pelvis extending down to thigh. Better in warm room. Especially indicated when menstrual pains are accompanied by vomiting and diarrhoea.

Worse · · Wet weather. After midnight. Cold or iced drinks. From food. Seashore. Right side.

Better — From heat. Head raised. Warm drinks.

Complementary: *Rhus tox., Carbo veg., Phos.*

Antidotes: *Carbo veg., China, Hepar sulph., Nux vom.*

Antidoted by: *Nux vom.,* Lime water.

Belladonna (Deadly Nightshade)

Belladonna is always associated with hot, red skin, flushed face, glaring eyes, throbbing carotids, excited mental state, restless sleep, delirium, convulsive movements, dryness of mouth and throat with aversion to water.

Characteristics: Nerve pains that come and go suddenly. Patient happy when well, but violent when sick. Starting or jumping out of bed. Child becomes very disobedient, will bite and slap parents' hands.

Patient often has hot head and cold hands and feet. Bullet-like pulse. Brain symptoms predominate. Fantastic rage. Destructive mania. Constant moanings. Acute local inflammation with sudden onset and rapid course. Sweat only on covered parts. Ailments predominantly right-handed. Acuteness of all senses. Likes sour things.

Sleeplessness. Patient is sleepy yet cannot sleep. Uneasy sleep before midnight. Child tosses and turns. Picks quarrels. Dry and hot to touch. Red face. Dilated pupils. Quick sensations. Imagines things, see ghosts, animals and hideous faces.

Headache. Headaches of great violence come on suddenly, last an indefinite time and depart suddenly. Violent throbbing in brain and carotids. Rush of blood to the head when lying. Bursting pain as if brain would be pressed out. Cutting knife stabs and shoots. Worse on stooping. Patient has vertigo, especially on rising and stooping. Tendency to fall to the left. Worse when wearing a hat. From light, motion and pressure.

Teething. One of the most important remedies in the teething of children. Red-hot face. Dry skin. Dilated pupils. Child twitches and fidgets. One of the useful remedies in toothache where the teeth have pus or holes in them. Violent pain starts while sleeping and relaxed.

Colds and Sore Throat. Dryness of mucous membranes. Suppressed catarrh with maddening headache. Snoring breathing and a danger of suffocation. Throat red, raw and sore, as if the inside is inflamed and swollen. Hurts to swallow. Ejection of food and drink through nose and mouth. Tongue is bright red. Inflammation starts on right side and moves to the left. Rapid progress.

Coughs. Dry cough, with dryness from larynx. Tickling and burning in larynx during violent spasm. Violent scraping in excited dry cough. Patient is red, burning hot, with dilated pupils. Peculiar cough; as soon as its great violence has raised a little mucus, the patient gets peace and stops coughing. Air passages grow drier and drier, begin to tickle, and then comes a spasm of coughing, as if all the air passages were taking part in it. The whoop and vomiting may follow, and therefore it is one of the great remedies for whooping cough. Child begins to cry immediately before cough comes on.

Intestinal Conditions. Abdominal pains are violent, come and disappear suddenly. Cramping pain. Violent pinchings. Tenderness of abdomen, made worse by slightest jar. Cannot bear slightest touch, even of bedclothes. Sensitive to pressure and draughts. Colic before stool and straining.

Fever. A high feverish state. Burning pungent steaming heat. Feet icy cold. Perspiration, dry only on head. No thirst with fever. An unquenchable craving for lemons and lemon juice. Remedy is rarely indicated when the whole body is sweating, or needs to be changed once the sweat sets in.

Convulsions. Useful remedy for convulsions. Patient strikes out and wants to escape.

Sunstroke. Temperature is high. Burning, restlessness. Onset is sudden. Vertigo. Nausea and vomiting. Frequent passing of urine, even when only a few drops have accumulated. Incontinence of urine and faeces. Congestion.

Menstruation. Menses increased, bright red, too early, too profuse. Foul smell. Dryness and heat in vagina and rectum. Sensation of forcing downwards or falling out.

Worse —   Summer sun, dry hot weather, heat, jar, touch, noise, draught, walking in wind, lying down, night after midnight, daytime after 3p.m., head getting wet, uncovered head, while drinking, while eating sausages.

Better —   Semi-erect. Warm room.

Compare: *Aconite, Bryonia, Gelsemium.*

Antidotes: *Camph., Coffea., Aconite., Opium.*

Complementary: *Calc.* Acute co-relative of *Calc. carb.*

Bryonia (Wild Hops)

An absolute 'must' for any medical chest.

Patient lies like a corpse, still and motionless. Resents being questioned. Inclined to be irritable and angry. Wants something, but it is hard to know what. Chilly, cannot sit up. Gets faint and sick. Has a confused brain. Wants to go home. Dreams of business. Onset of trouble is slow, often after constipation. It is a very deep-seated remedy, and acts on all fibrous tissues. Is useful in acute conditions like sinusitis, etc., but is rarely indicated for earache, tonsilitis, and very rarely for kidney colic.

Headache. Bursting, splitting headache. Vertigo, nausea, faintness on rising, or sitting up. Rush of blood to the head. Feels as if hit with a hammer from inside. Worse from slightest movement. Worse after washing with cold water. Irritable. Thirsty. Dry lips and mouth. Face sweaty.

Sleeplessness. Restless, can only sleep for half an hour. When slumbering is continually thinking about what he has read the previous evening. Thirst. Heat. Frequent shivering sensations of one arm or foot, then sweat. Illusion of being away from home, and wants to go home.

Nose Bleed. Frequent bleeding of nose when menses should appear. Also in morning, relieving headache.

Colds and Coughs. Cold begins with sneezing and running of the nose. Coryza. Running of the eyes, with aching eyes and body. Cold then goes to the throat and larynx, with hoarseness, and travels down into the lungs, with bronchitis. Dry spasmodic cough. Cough shakes whole body. Very little expectoration. Worse at night, on entering a warm room, after eating or drinking. Thirsty for cold drinks. Irritable. Patient sleeps and sleeps, and wants to be left alone. Lips hard and dry. Headache as if the head will fly to pieces. Cough worse on taking a deep breath.

Digestive Disorders. Pressure in stomach after eating, as though a stone is lying there and making him cross. Stomach extremely sensitive to touch and pressure. Vomiting of bile. Mouth is dry, tongue white. Thirst for large quantities at long intervals. Patient cannot bear disturbance of any kind, mental or physical. Severe headache.

Unnatural hunger or loss of appetite. Desire for acid, sweets, oysters. Vomiting of bile and water immediately after eating or drinking, especially of warm drinks. Stools hard and dry as if burnt, seem too large. No desire, or urging with several attempts before result, which is then unsatisfactory.

Abdominal Colic. Patient lies still, and keeps his knees up to relax abdominal muscles. Is unable to move. Does not want to walk, or think. Diarrhoea preceded by cutting pain in abdomen.

Menstruation. Irregular menstruation. Splitting headache. Pain in breasts, must be supported. Frequent nose bleeding at start of menses. Pain with abdominal and pelvic soreness.

Influenza (Breakbone fever). Wants to lie still, and be left alone. Anxiety, dreams and delirium are of business. Internal heat. Easy, profuse perspiration. Pulse hard, tense and quick. Thirst for cold drinks. Worse from every movement and noise. Chill with external coldness, dry cough, stitches.

Worse — Hot weather. Morning. Warmth. Any motion. Exertion. Touch. Cannot sit up, gets faint and sick.

Better — Cold things. Lying on painful side. Rest. Pressure.
Complementary: *Rhus tox., Alumina.*
Antidotes: *Aconite, Chamomilla, Nux vomica.*
Compare: *Kali mur., Ptelae.*

Calcarea carbonica (Oyster shell)
Characteristics: The oyster forms a shell and builds. The patient is an oyster without a shell and is unprotected. Usually fair. State of fear, fear of losing reason, or that people will observe his mental confusion. Runs into the dark. Doubts his health ('How is my heart?'). Comes to the doctor to gain confidence. Difficult to work with. Desires to be magnetized. Children irritable, peevish, obstinate and lazy. Child likes to eat anything — lead, coal, wood and pencils. Adult craves eggs, chalk and indigestible things. Chilly. Dizzy. Easy sweating of single parts, e.g. the head wetting the pillow when asleep. Longing for fresh air, which inspires, benefits and strengthens. Feels better in every way when constipated.

Adults — Dilated pupils. Colds go to the chest and are caught easily. Head feels internally and externally cold. Painless hoarseness, worse in the morning. Hyper-acidic sour stomach. Stool has to be removed mechanically. Menstruation is too early, too profuse and long lasting, and least mental excitement causes an increased return of menstrual flow.

Children — Late teething (sitting up and walking before teeth arrive). Decaying teeth. Large-sized head and/or stomach. Bow legs, rickets, weak back, muscular weakness. Feet habitually cold, as if child had cold damp socks on. Continually cold in bed. Specially indicated when child has suffered from several acute Belladonna troubles. Great liability to catch colds.

NOTE: In aged people it should not be repeated, especially if first dose benefited. If repeated it will do harm.

Complementary to *Belladonna*, which is the acute of *Calcarea*. Acts best before *Lyco., Nux. phos., Silica.*

Calcarea phosphorica
Characteristics: The perfect cosmopolitan. A dark skinny edition of *Calc. carb.* with a tendency to grow too fast and too slender. Changeable; desires to be in different places. Memory weak, writes

wrong words. Screams easily. Involuntary sighing. Feels complaints more when thinking of them. Wants all kinds of salty things. Very large cervical glands. Swollen tonsils. The neck flops and the head is too heavy. Slow teething, teething problems in skinny dark babies. Headaches and backaches in schoolgirls. Coughs in girls at puberty, who grow too fast. Tendency to grow too fast and too slender. Sprains of the ankle. Non-union of fractures — give two or three weeks to promote union. (*Symphytum* for first two days and then *Calc. phos.*).

At every attempt to eat, colic pains occur in the abdomen. Useful for polypi, piles, if not bleeding badly. Ailments from grief, from disappointed love.
Complementary: *Ruta.*

Calendula officinalis (Marigold)
A most remarkable healing agent: applied locally. Useful for washing cuts and open wounds, parts that will not heal and ulcers. Useful for dressing infected cuts. Prevents infections of wounds. Is useful in old neglected wounds threatening gangrene. Useful in ulcers of various kinds, and in excessive discharge of pus. Exhaustion from loss of blood. Excessive pain as if having been beaten. Compound fractures. It is most often used locally in the form of fluid extract, but is extremely useful internally by mouth particularly in healing clean wounds from operations or knife cuts, etc.

Coughs and Colds. Nose blocked on one side and coryza on the other. Green pus. Cough with green expectoration. Hoarseness.

Fever. Coldness, with great sensitivity to open air. Heat in the evening.

Burns. Useful for superficial burns and scalds.
Worse — In damp, heavy, cloudy weather.
Compare: *Hamamelis, Hypericum, Arnica, Symphytum.*
Antidotes: *Chelidon, Rheum.*
Complementary: *Hepar sulph.*

Carbo vegetabilis (Vegetable Charcoal)
Characteristics: The typical *Carbo* patient is faint, weak, cold, blue, at the peripheral. Mentally sluggish, weak and slow. Memory weak. Aversion to darkness. Fear of ghosts. Patient may be almost lifeless, but head is hot. Must have fresh air, wishes to be fanned, must have all the windows open. Very debilitated. Pulse imperceptible, oppressed

and quickened respiration. Faints easily, and is worn out. Slow venous circulation. Tip of nose inclined to be reddish-blue, like all peripheral parts.

Headache. Aches from any over-indulgence. Head feels heavy and constricted. Hat upon head feels like a heavy weight. Vertigo with nausea.

Coughs and Colds. Worse in warm moist weather. Coryza catarrhal inflammation of nose with cough. Raw throat. Loses his voice every evening. Dry tickling cough. Ineffectual efforts to sneeze. Burning in chest as from glowing coals. Cold breath and sweat. Cold mouth and tongue. Bronchitis. Patient collapsed, 'almost gone' sensation. For this sensation in any illness, *Carbo veg.* is a very useful remedy.

Whooping Cough. Useful remedy in early stages. Cough wild, hard, rough. Every violent spell of coughing brings up a lump of phlegm, or is followed by retching, choking and vomiting. Pain in chest after cough. Redness of face. Craving for salt.

Digestive System. Excessive flatulence. Food decomposes in the stomach; weak digestion, simplest food disagrees. Excessive accumulation of gas in the stomach and intestines. Worse lying down and after eating and drinking. Burning feeling in stomach, which feels distended and as if it would burst. Better for loosening clothes. Effects of debauch, late suppers and rich food. Bitter salty taste in mouth. Gas travels upwards. Better passing wind.

Diarrhoea. Frequent, involuntary, cadaverous smelling stools, followed by burning. Soft stool voided with difficulty. Patient's face pale or greenish. Skin damp and cold. Tongue and breath cold. Burning in rectum.

Menstruation. Pain starts before menstruation begins, accompanied by cold clammy sensations. Better from fresh air. Menstrual pains accompanied by thick black clots or cold clammy sweats, as if faint.

Worse — Warm damp weather. Evening, night and open air. Cold. From fat food, butter, coffee.

Better — From cold applications. Fanning. Belching. Quiet belching (better belching and bearing the shame, than stopping and bearing the pain).

Complementary: *Kali carb., Phos., Puls.*

Compare: *Lycop., China.*

Antidotes: *Nux vomica, Camph., Ars. alb.*

Causticum (Mixture of *Ammonium* and *Kali natrum* group)
Characteristics: Dark-haired, rigid, weak persons, with excessively yellow and sallow complexions. Not self-reliant. Intensely sympathetic. Sudden emotions. Anxious. Worse in the evening. Weak memories. Absent-mindedness. Mental labour causes tightness of scalp. Dizziness, with fear of falling. Children do not want to go to bed at night. Right-sided remedy. Chronic, rheumatic, arthritic and paralytic affections, indicated by tearing and drawing pains in the muscular and fibrous tissues, with deformities about the joints. Rawness and soreness of various parts. Bruised muscular pain in neck, back and coccyx.

Eyes. Dim vision as if looking through a cloud of insects. Acute or chronic drooping of the upper lids which feel as if they are sticking to the lower. Sudden fleeting loss of sight.

Ears. Rushing and roaring sound in the ear. His own sounds echo in his ears. Colds extend to his ears.

Colds and Coughs. Nasal discharge thick and yellow, with sore inside of nose. Dry tickling cough, hoarseness, better for cold drink. Throat, although it feels raw and scraped, is painless. Cough is loose, but difficult to get up. Sputum slips back. Painless loss of voice. Paralysis of vocal chords.

Urine. Sudden urge to void, and he has to rush or have an accident, and yet has to wait for a while before the flow starts.

Menstruation. Menses only during day, too early, too feeble. Ceases on lying down.
Better — In damp wet weather.
Worse — In clear fine weather. In cold air.
Compare: *Arn., Gels., Sepia, Rumex, Carbo veg.*
Complementary: *Carbo veg., Petros.*
Incompatible: Must not be used after or before *Phos.* and *Coffea.*

Chamomilla (German Chamomile)
The chief symptoms belong to the mental and emotional group, which leads us to this remedy in many forms of disease.

Characteristics: Spiteful, uncivil, irritable, over-sensitive. Unable to bear pain. Pain becomes intolerable at night causing patient to jump out of bed, and walk about. Child peevish, nothing pleases. Always complaining. Moans because he cannot have what he wants. Quiet only when carried, needs petting constantly. Can have convulsions after a fit of anger. Thirsty, hot, numb. Sensitive to high winds, especially about his ears.

Sleeplessness. Sleepy, but cannot sleep. Restless. Drowsiness with moaning, weeping and wailing during sleep. If he sits down during the day he wishes to sleep, but if he lies down he can't sleep. Anxious, frightened dreams. Starts out of sleep and becomes cross and ugly.

Headache. Throbbing in one half of the brain. Inclined to bend head backwards. Hot clammy seat on forehead and scalp.

Earache. Ringing in ears. Earache, with soreness and heat, driving patient frantic. One cheek flushed and hot, the other pale and cold. Stitching pain. Ears feel stopped. Discharge with soreness.

Toothache. Pain if anything warm is taken.

Coughs. Hard dry cough. Coughs in sleep. Coughs when angry. Impatient of suffering, irritable, capricious. One cheek flushed.

Stomach and Digestion. Putrid breath after meals. Distended. Bilious vomiting. Nausea after coffee. Aversion to warm drinks. Tongue yellow. Bitter taste. Acid rises in throat. Shivers in cold air. One cheek red. Tearing pain in abdomen. Restless.

Intestinal Conditions. Violent retching. Covered with cold sweat. Cutting colic. Diarrhoea with colic. Doubles up and screams. White and slimy or pale green watery diarrhoea. Stools hot, smelling of rotten eggs. Excessive sensibility to pain, especially in teething babies.

Menstruation. Profuse discharge with labour-like pains. Pains spasmodic. Patient intolerant to pain.

Worse — From heat. Anger. Evening. Before midnight. Open air. In the wind. Eructations.

Better — Warm, wet weather. Fasting.

Compare: *Belladonna, Bryonia, Coffea, Pulsatilla, Sulphur.*

Complementary: *Belladonna, Mag. phos.*

Chamomilla is swift acting, but not a very searching remedy.

Chelidonium (Celandine)

A very ancient liver remedy.

Characteristics: Thin fair complexion subjects. Despondent, depressed, sad, anxious, brooding, weepy, pessimistic. Tendency to gastric and liver complaints. General lethargy and indisposition to make any effort. Bilious complication during pregnancy. Ailments brought on and renewed by change of weather. Right-sided. Bloated.

Headache. Heavy, lethargic, drowsy. Head feels as heavy as lead. Vertigo, associated with liver disturbance. Remedy for hangover when you cannot even begin to get up.

Stomach. Main gastric symptoms are of nausea and vomiting. Pain through stomach to back and right shoulder blade. Dizziness improved by vomiting. Patient better from heat. Vomiting by eating which gives temporary relief. Desires hot drinks. Dislikes cheese.
   Chest conditions, especially asthma, occur only at night.
Worse —   Change of weather. Warmth. 4 a.m. and at 4 p.m. Early in the morning. Right side. Motion. Touch.
Better —   After eating. From pressure.
Complementary: *Bryonia, Lycop.*
Compare: *Nux vom., Sulph., Bryonia, Ars.*

Dioscorea villosa (Wild Yam)
A useful remedy for stomach pain.

Characteristics: Deep abdominal discomfort. Patient is doubled up with acute pain. Belching of large quantities of offensive gas. Sinking feeling in the pit of stomach. Neuralgia of the stomach. Pain along the breast bone. Cutting pains radiate to the chest and arms when bending forward and while lying down. Sharp pain in pit of stomach relieved by standing erect. Pains suddenly shift to different parts, and appear in remote localities. Sharp pains from liver shoot upwards to right nipple.
Worse —   Evening and night. Lying down and doubling up.
Better —   Standing erect. Motion in open air. Pressure.
   The remedy should not be used before or after *Chamomile* or *Camphor.*
   It compares well with *Nux vomica* and *Bryonia.*

Drosera (Sun-dew)
Queen of whooping coughs. Coldness of left half of face, with stinging pains and dry heat in right half. Measles with spasmodic cough. Glands of neck enlarged.

Cough. Spasmodic, dry irritating cough, with violent paroxysms which follow each other so rapidly that breathing becomes impossible. Choking occurs, patient gets cold and clammy and vomits. Coughs with yellow expectoration, with bleeding from nose and mouth. Coughs worse after midnight, warmth, drinking, singing, laughing, lying down.

Clergyman's sore throat, with rough scraping, dry sensation deep in the throat, hoarse voice, which is toneless, cracked and requires exertion to produce.

NOTE: One single dose of the 30th potency is sufficient to cure epidemic whooping cough. The cure takes place between the seventh and eighth day. Do not give another dose immediately after the first, as it will not only prevent the good effect of the former, but will also be injurious. (Hahnemann's *Materia Medica Pura*.)
Compare: *Cina, Corallium, Cuprum, Ipecac, Sambucus.*
Complementary: *Nux vom.*
Follows well after *Sambucus, Sulphur, Veratrum.*
Is well followed by *Calcarea, Pulsatilla, Sulphur.*

Eupatorium (Thoroughwort)
Known as 'Bone-set' from the prompt manner in which it relieves pain in limbs and muscles accompanying fevers like influenza and malaria. Sluggishness in all organs and functions, and patient feels worn out, often with bilious or breakbone fevers.

Influenza, Malaria and such Fevers. Bruised soreness and chills running up the back. Feeling as if the body is broken all over. Perspiration relieves all symptoms except headache. Chill between 7 a.m. and 9 a.m. preceded by thirst with great soreness and aching of the bones. Throbbing headache. Nausea and vomiting of bile between chilly and hot stage. Extremely thirsty during a chill only. Nausea.
Worse —   Odours of food. Periodically. 7-9 a.m.
Better —   From conversation, and getting on hands and knees.
Compare: *Bryonia, Chel., Ars. alb., Nat. mur., Phos., Acid.*

Loss of weight and energy is very rapid, and sometimes within a couple of days.

Morning hoarseness with bruised soreness in chest.

NOTE: *Bryonia* is the nearest remedy in influenza but it has free sweating with pain which keeps the patient still, while *Eup.* sweats scantily and is restless with pain.

Ferrum phosphoricum (Phosphate of Iron)
Grauvogl's Oxygenoid Constitution. Worse for cold, and yet better for cold applications. Aversion to meat and milk. Desire for stimulants. Useful for ill-effects of sun and heat. Complaints from taking cold or suppressed perspiration. Articular rheumatism, with fever and shooting pains worse for movement, and yet better for gentle motion. Child loves being in a cradle. Worse 4-6 a.m. and 4-6 p.m.

Headache. Better for cold applications.

Blood. Haemorrhages from any outlet, of bright red blood. Anaemia with easy flushings of the face. Passive, congested and bleeding.

Abdomen. First stages of dysentery, with blood in discharges. Urine spurts with every cough. Incontinence. Enuresis.

Fever. Chill every day at 1 p.m.

Menstruation. Menses every three weeks, with bearing down sensation, and pain on the top of the head. Vagina dry and hot.
Better — Gentle movement. Cold applications.
Worse — At night, 4-6 a.m. On right side. From touch. Jar. Motion in general.
Compare: *Aconite, Gels., China, Ars., Graph., Petroleum.*

Gelsemium (Yellow Jasmine)
Characteristics: The patient is mentally and physically relaxed. Very weak; powerless, numb, drowsy, has a fever without thirst and wishes to be left alone. May have a desire to throw himself from a height with absolute lack of fear. Lies sleepless, languid but cannot compose the mind. Delirious on falling asleep. Emotional excitement leading to bodily ailments. Bad effects from fear or exciting news. Stage fright. Child starts suddenly and grasps the nurse. Screams as if he is afraid of falling. Neurotic hysterical subjects, especially women and children. Nervous symptoms predominate in all complaints. There may be a desire for expression in speech or writing with increased sense of power. Tingling or coldness of affected parts. Passive congestion. Heaviness and paralytic feeling. Hot head and cold extremities. Dusky red face. Drooping eyelids. Chill up and down the back. Involuntary stools, or frequent urination from fright or anticipation of an ordeal. Profuse urination. Actors funk or examination funk where the nervousness starts even before preparation begins. Nervousness with a deep sense of inadequacy, not supported by intelligence.

Headache. Dull headache with fever. Dull tired ache at base of brain, or beginning at the nape of the neck, and extending overhead to one eye, generally the right eye, sometimes both eyes. Headache commences with blurred vision, and accompanied by vertigo. Relieved by profuse urination.

Colds. Sneezing and catarrh, with a watery mucous discharge. Much sneezing early morning. Nostrils sore, as if hot water passing through them. *Gelsemium* suits colds and fevers of mild winters. Chills up and down the back. Tiredness of the whole body. Better near the fire.

Sore Throat. Difficulty in swallowing, especially warm food. Tonsils swollen. Throat feels rough and burning. Shooting pain in ears, all swallowing causes pain in ears. Shuddering as if ice rubbed up back. High temperature. Hot skin. Cold extremities. Heaviness and tiredness of whole body. Patient worse in damp weather and before a thunderstorm. Worse before emotion, excitement, or bad news, or in thinking of his ailments. Better bending forward. Better in open air, continual motion, profuse urination, and with stimulants.

Influenza. Wants to be held because he shakes so much. Pulse slow, full, soft. Chilliness up and down back. Heat and sweat stages long and exhausting. Muscular soreness, great prostration and violent headache.

Worse —   Damp weather. Fog. Before a thunderstorm. Emotion. Excitement. Bad news. Tobacco smoking. When thinking of his ailments.

Better —   In open air. Continued motion. Bending forward. By profuse urination. Stimulants.

Compare: *Ignatia, Baptisia, Aconite, Belladonna, Mag. phos.*
Antidotes: *China, Coffea.*
Alcoholic stimulants relieve all complaints where *Gelsemium* is useful.

Hepar sulphuris calcarea (Hahnemann's Calcium Sulphide)
Characteristics: Plump, chubby, lymphatic, slow, inactive, irritable, violent, critical, swearing, great sensitiveness to all impressions. Becomes offended very easily. Outwardly calm, but inwardly extremely restless and active. Trifles make him angry, and his resentments are fierce. Hates being touched. Sweating patient pulls blankets around him. Chilly. Will wear overcoat even in hot weather. Hypersensitive. Cannot bear pain. General sourness of all excretions. Profuse and easy sweating. Unhealthy skin. Everything suppurates.

In the beginning of an abscess it hastens the formation of pus and points it in the safest direction for the body. Patient is better in himself for eating but worse in his stomach. Desires vinegar, sour and pungent things, and fat.

Eyes. Useful in superficial ulcers of the eyes. Conjunctivitis.

Throat. Sensation of splinter or stitching pains.

Cough. Weakness and much rattling in the chest. Croupy, choking, strangling cough. Worse on any part of the body being exposed or uncovered, from any exposure to dry cold wind, cold air, cold drinks, and before midnight or towards morning.

Skin. Unhealthy skin, with every little injury suppurating. Skin very sensitive to touch. Very sensitive ulcers. Patient cannot bear even clothes to touch affected parts. Skin affections are extremely sensitive and therefore patient may faint when ulcers or pimples are touched for dressing. Chapped skin with dry cracks on hands and feet. Useful remedy for injuries to the nail. Also suitable for infections.

NOTE: In inflammation, a careful consideration of the stages would help either abortion of the inflammation, or hasten suppuration. A high potency in a single dose helps to abort if pus has not already formed; while low potencies in repeated doses would hasten suppuration and discharge an abscess which has pus already. You should consult the doctor before taking a high potency.

Better — For warmth, wrapping up, damp warm weather, especially the head. Better in himself for eating but worse in his stomach.

Worse — At night, lying on painful side, in slightest draught, uncovering, eating or drinking cold things, perspiring, from touch, from cold, cold air, from wind.

Complementary to *Calendula* in injuries to soft parts.

Calc. carb. follows well.

Compare: *Aconite, Staphysagria, Silica, Spongia.*

Antidotes: Mercury and other metals, iodine, iodine of potassium.

When taking *Hepar sulph.,* do not take coffee.

Hypericum (St John's Wort)

Great remedy for injuries to the nerves, especially fingers and toes. Crushed finger tips. Foreign body in the nail. Excessive painfulness is a guiding symptom to its use. Punctured, incised or lacerated wounds, especially in parts rich in nerves. Intense pain and soreness. Injuries from splinters or treading on a nail. It prevents tetanus. Relieves pain after operations, in fact, supersedes morphia. Constant drowsiness. Patient desires wine, warm drinks and has a great thirst.

Shock. Bad effects of brain or spinal concussion where there is severe nerve injury. Constant drowsiness.

Headache. Pain of neuralgia type. Dull ache. Heavy, feels as if touched by an icy cold hand. Brain seems compressed. Head feels long. Sensation of being lifted high in the air. Melancholy.

Toothache. Nerve pain in the tooth of a pulling, tearing character. Also nerve-root pains after extraction of teeth.

Abdomen and Stomach. Diarrhoea due to sun and overheating in the summer. Loose yellow stools. Thirst, nausea. Tongue coated white at base, tip clean. Feeling of lump in stomach.

Haemorrhoids. Piles with pain, bleeding and tenderness. Driving dull urging pain in rectum (Nerve pain).

Menstruation. Too late, accompanied by headache and aching pain in abdomen.

Injuries. Piercing wounds from sharp instruments. Injuries to spine and coccyx, with pain radiating up spine and down limbs.

Punctured wounds, dog, cat and rat bites are made safe and heal rapidly by Ledum, but if the pain shoots up the nerve, *Hypericum* is the indicated remedy.

Worse — In cold, dampness, foggy weather; in the warm; from touch and least exposure.

Better — Head bent backwards.

Compare: *Ledum, Arnica, Calendula, Ruta, Coff.*

Antidotes: *Ars., Chamomilla.*

Can be alternated with *Arnica.*

Ignatia (St Ignatius Bean)

Characteristics: The *Ignatia* type takes life and duties seriously. The emotional element is uppermost, and co-ordination of function is interfered with. One of the best remedies for hysteria. Especially adapted to the nervous temperament. Women of sensitive, easily excited nature. Often melancholic, sad, tearful. Mental and physical exhaustion after long concentrated grief. Rapidly alternating moods.

Unable to control themselves, because they cannot collect themselves. Easily crying out. Weeping in silence, sitting and sighing. Better alone, but do not resent consolation. Nervous, hysterical, mild disposition. Comparatively unselfish. Quick to perceive, rapid in execution. An Astral person, full of paradoxes, falls in love when nothing can come of it (lady in love with the coachman).

Sore throat, better for eating rough food. Pain on swallowing nothing, no pain on swallowing food. Thirst during chill, no thirst during fever. Cough better for coughing. Roaring in ears, better for hearing music. Indigestion, better for eating. Empty feeling in stomach, not better for eating. Spasmodic laughter from grief. Colour of face changes when addressed. Sweat on the face in a small spot, only while eating. Chilly person, but likes cold food. Violent aversion to tobacco and fumes of tobacco. Does not enjoy his normal tobacco. Dislikes stimulants and yet feels the need. Craves sour things. Chilly person. Pains better for heat (except stomach pains which are better for cold food). Complaints return at precisely the same hour.

Shock. One of the important remedies for shock, especially if caused by fright, grief or fear. Useful remedy for hysterics and fainting if caused by grief or mental shock, bad news or a psychological cause. Globus hystericus, difficult swallowing. Hysterical paralysis, loss of voice, hearing.

Headache. Boring pain, as if head is being drilled.

Eyes. Flashes and flickerings of light in the eyes, both generally and particularly, which are better when patient eats.

Chest. Dry spasmodic cough.

Stomach. Pain, better for cold food.

Rectum. Rectal spasm, excessively painful and ineffectual. Constipation very much affected by emotion and excitement. Tendency to haemorrhoids and prolapse. Sharp stitches shoot up the rectum. Fissure, even in a patient who is not constipated.

Fever. Red face during chill, thirst during chill only. Heat without thirst. Better external heat, worse for covering.

Worse — In the morning, in open air, after meals, coffee, smoking, liquids, external warmth.

Better — While eating, change of position.

Compare: *Kali phos.*

Complementary: *Ars., Nat. mur., Phos.*

Incompatible: *Coffea, Tabac.*
Antidotes:*Puls., Nux., Cham.*
When taking *Ignatia* do not take coffee.

Kali bichromicum (Potassium Bichromate)

Characteristics: This remedy is specially indicated for fat fleshy people with light complexions, subject to catarrh and stringy discharges. Symptoms are worse in the morning. Pains wander about, appear and disappear suddenly. Very weak memory, listless, languid, indisposed to mental and physical work. Sleep terminates between 3 and 4 a.m.

Headache. Vertigo and headaches. Worse on rising from sitting or lying position. Headache in the scalp. Better by pressure, open air, eating; worse from stroking motion, lying on it at night.

Eyes. Pain above the eyes, worse on right side. Eyelids swollen, burning, oedematous, sometimes with stringy mucoid discharge.

Ears. Thick yellow discharge from ears, both sides. Swelling in the ears with sharp stitching, pinpoint pains, hurts.

Sore Throat. Throat trouble with shooting pain extending to the ear. Tonsils swollen and inflamed. Parotid glands swollen. Uvula relaxed. Throat dry and rough.

Colds. Pressure and pain at root of nose. Discharge thick, ropy, greenish-yellow and offensive. Mucus can be drawn out in long strands. Dryness in nose. Coryza with obstruction of nose. Loss of smell. Violent sneezing. Inability to breathe through nose. Snuffles of children, especially fat, chubby babies. Ulcerations of mucous membrane.

Coughs. Voice hoarse, worse in the evening. Tickling in larynx. Cough is with white mucus, that can be drawn out in strings. Cough with pain in sternum. Hoarseness, metallic cough, breathlessness, worse lying down.

Intestinal Condition. Averse to meat. Desires acids, lemons, etc. and beer which does not agree. Nausea, vomiting of burning mucus — stringy vomiting. Diarrhoea, with stringy mucous discharge.

Menses. Painful, too soon, with headaches. Vertigo, feverishness and nausea. Leucorrhoea yellow ropy, can be drawn out in long strings — Tenacious mucus.

Pains. Are pinpointed. Patient localizes a small area exactly and the pains shift rapidly from place to place — appear and disappear suddenly. Rheumatic pains alternate with gastric complaints. Worse in autumn and the digestion worse in spring.

Skin. Hot, red, dry skin with dry eruptions and small pustules over whole body. Worse in cold weather.

Nose, throat and bladder all partake of the catarrhal condition. *Kali bich.* can be used in measles.

Better — From heat and applications of heat.

Worse — Beer, morning, hot weather, undressing.

Compare: *Brom., Hepar, Calc. sulph., Ac., Ipecac.*

Antidotes: *Ars., Lach., Pulsatilla.*

Antimonium tart. follows well after affection of catarrhal type and skin disorders.

Potassium *kali* remedies are not indicated where there is fever, and they do not bear frequent repetition.

Kali carbonicum (Carbonate of Potassium)

Characteristics: Fat and flabby people. Soft pulse, coldness and general depression. Mentally and physically lethargic. Easily frightened. Easily worried about the future. Sensitive to noise, touch and pain. Alternating moods. Very irritable. Never wants to be left alone. Never quiet or contented. Anxiety felt in stomach. Sensation as if bed were sinking. Early morning aggravation is very characteristic. Sensitive to every change of atmosphere and intolerance of cold. Right-sided ailments. Pinpointed pains.

Headache. Vertigo on turning. Headache from riding in cold wind. Pain comes on with yawning. Stitches in temple, one-sided. Nausea.

Eyes. Stitches in eyes. Lids stick together in morning. Swelling over upper lid, like little bags.

Colds and Coughs. Catarrhal condition of all mucous membranes, with a feeling of dryness. Thick, fluent yellow discharge. Tenacious mucus or pus which must be swallowed, resulting in choking or vomiting. Nose stuffs up in warm room. Catches cold with every exposure to fresh air.

Hoarseness. Loss of voice. Feels as if lump in throat that must be swallowed. Stinging pain when swallowing. Stiff neck. Chilliness. Fish-bone sensation in throat as soon as he becomes cold. Sputum of small round lumps of blood-streaked mucus. Perspires much. Cheesy taste. Worse in cold air and draughts. Dry hard cough, worse at 3 a.m. Throat dry, rough and parched. Better for warmth.

Indicated for croupy, spasmodic coughs and therefore one of the useful remedies in whooping cough.

Stomach. Flatulence. Capricious appetite, with strong desire for sweet things. Feeling of lump in pit of stomach. Disgust for food. Nausea, better lying down. Sour vomiting. Constant feeling as if stomach were full of water. Chokes easily when eating. Cutting feeling in intestines, must sit bent over pressing body with hands, or lean far back for relief.

Menstruation. Weakness and sadness before menses. Backache, and wants back pressed. Pain similar to labour pains. Patient feels unwell. Compare: *Bry.*, *Lyco.*, *Nat. mur.*, *Nit. Acid.*, *Stannum.*
Complementary: *Carbo* (very often administration of *Carbo veg.* or *Nux vomica* beforehand will help a patient and make him sensitive to *Kali carb.*)
Antidotes: *Camph.*, *Coffea.*

Kali phosphoricum (Phosphate of Potassium)
Characteristics: One of the greatest nerve remedies. Weakness and tiredness. Specially adapted to the young. Marked disturbance of the sympathetic nervous system. Conditions arising from want of nerve power. Mental and physical depression is wonderfully improved by this remedy. Causes are usually excitement, overwork and worry. Mental characteristics are anxiety, nervous strain, lethargy, indisposition to meet people. Very nervous, starts easily. Irritable. Nightmares. Loss of memory. Brain fag. Great despondency.

Headache. Headaches with 'empty gone' sensation in stomach. Vertigo. Relieved by gentle movement. Headache of students and those worn out by fatigue. Loss of perceptive powers. Humming and buzzing in the ear.

Toothaches with bleeding gums. Spongy receding gums.

Coughs with yellow phlegm, low temperature and increases after food.

Stomach. A nervous 'gone' sensation in pit of stomach. Seasick without nausea. Diarrhoea occasioned by fright. Better for warmth and rest. Worse while eating.

Influenza. Post-influenzal debilities.

General weakness and gloom.

Worse — Excitement, worry, mental and physical exertion, eating, cold, early morning.

Better — Warmth, rest, nourishment, affection.

Magnesia phosphorica (Phosphate of Magnesia)

The great anti-spasmodic remedy. Specially suited to dark, thin, highly nervous, tired, languid, exhausted subjects.

Characteristics: Indisposition for mental exertion. Sharp cutting, stabbing neuralgic pains almost unbearable, driving patient crazy. Pains change place rapidly. Relieved by warmth. Great dread of cold air and uncovering. Laments all the time about the pain. Inability to think clearly.

Headache. Pain after mental labour, with chilliness. Headaches in school girls, face red, flushed with emotion. Vertigo on moving, falls forward on closing eyes. Worse between 10 and 11 a.m., or 4 and 5 p.m. Better for pressure and warmth.

Ears. Severe neuralgic pains. Worse behind right ear. Worse by going into the cold air, and washing face and neck with cold water.

Toothache. Pain better by heat and hot liquids. Ulceration of teeth, with swelling of glands of face, throat and neck. Complaints of teething in children.

Digestive System, Stomach, Abdomen. Cramping neuralgic pains of stomach, abdomen and pelvis. Complaints from standing in cold water or working in cold clay. Colic and flatulence, forcing patient to bend double. Relieved by rubbing, warmth, pressure. Accompanied by belching of gas, which gives no relief.

Hiccups, with retching day and night. Thirst for cold drinks. Bloated sensation in abdomen. Must loosen clothing, walk about and pass wind. Constipation in rheumatic subjects due to flatulence and indigestion.

Menstuation. Menstrual colic. Menses too early, dark, stringy. Darting pains. Worse before but better when flow starts. Worse on right side. Better by heat and bending double. Swelling of external parts.

Worse — Right side. Cold. Touch. At night.

Better — Warmth. Bending double. Pressure. Friction.

Compare: *Kali phos., Colocy, Silica, Zinc, Dioscorea.*
Antidotes: *Belladonna, Gelsemium, Lachesis.*

Mercurius (Quicksilver)

Characteristics: Light-haired type of person. Lax muscle and skin conditions. Great weakness and trembling. Slow in answering questions. Weak memory. Loss of will power. Mistrustful. Weary of life. Thinks he is losing his reason. Sensitive to heat and cold. Anxious, restless, tossing about, moving from place to place. Irritable. Hurried and rapid talking. Aching pains in joints. Oily offensive perspiration.

Eyes. Almost magic remedy for severe aching pains behind the eyeballs. Lids red and swollen. Profuse acrid discharge. Worse after exposure to the glare of fire.

Ears. Pain in ears worse from warmth of bed. Yellow discharge, heated and bloody. Oil in external canal.

Headache. Head congested, feels as if it will burst. Fullness of brain. Head feels as if in a vice. Burning, especially of left temple. Pain over nose and eyes. Feels as if tied by something tight. Wants to be covered but worse for heat. Perspiration of head oily and offensive. Sensitive to air.

Nose. Coryza, with acrid discharge. Copious discharge of corroding mucus. Raw smarting sensation. Much sneezing. Sneezing in sunshine. Nostrils ulcerated. Worse in damp weather.

Throat. Ulcers and inflammation appearing at every change of weather. Constant desire to swallow. Stitches into ear on swallowing. Fluids return through nose. More difficult to swallow liquids than solids. Complete loss of voice. Burning in throat as if from hot vapour ascending. Uvula often swollen, dark and red. Any attempt to swallow causes violent spasm in throat with ejection of solids or liquids. Distinguished from *Belladonna* by its intense destructive inflammation of throat.

Mouth and Throat. Every little exposure to a damp atmosphere causes catarrh and coryza. Disagreeable odour of breath with metallic taste — both, although difficult to describe, are characteristic.

Cough. Expectoration of virulent yellow mucus. Catarrh. Paroxysms worse at night, and from warmth of bed. Chilliness. Dread of air.

Stitches from lower part of right lung to back. Cough worse by inhaling tobacco smoke. Cannot bear smoking, or anyone else to smoke near them. Worse in damp weather, lying on right side, in warm room, in warm bed. Tendency to perspire, but no better for it.

Diarrhoea. Peculiar bruised sensation about the sacrum. Tender to touch. Painful bloody discharge with vomiting, often without reason, and sometimes mouth gets filled up with saliva for no apparent reason. Nothing passed except mucus tinged with blood. Diarrhoea, with terrible straining before, with and after stool. Very distressing tinesmus. Persistent cutting colic pains. Discharge accompanied by chilliness. Never-get-done feeling.

Be very careful in the choice between *Mercurius* and *Silica*. *Mercurius* must never be taken before, with or after *Silica*.

Skin. Constant sweating, often oily, with no relief from sweating. Debilitating sweats worse at night. Itching, worse from warmth of bed. Yellowish-brown crust formed over the scalp and skin with thick foul smelling discharge.

Worse — Damp weather. At night. In a warm room. A warm bed. Lying on the right side. Perspiring. Motion. Bone pains and rheumatic conditions are markedly worse at night.

Compare: *Mez., Phos., Syph., Kali mur.*

Antidote: *Hep., Aur., Mez.*

Complementary: *Badiaga.*

Although quicksilver or *Merc. vivus* and *Merc. sol.* (Hahnemann) provings have been given separately by some authorities, others have treated them as similar and synonymous. In the search through the history of their provings, it was found that most provings have been chosen from the history of the allopathic administration of massive doses of *Merc.* in the past. I have therefore always considered them as one.

Inflammation just before suppuration anywhere, such as throat, whitlow, etc. draws attention to this remedy. Throat is bright red and swollen and has difficulty in swallowing fluids. This kind of swollen pain with narrowing of tracts is a particular indication. It is indicated therefore in cases where there is a need to evacuate pus.

Natrum muriaticum (Chloride of Sodium)
Characteristics: A dull absent-minded person, with a weak memory, who has difficulty in thinking. Likes to dwell on past disagreeable occurrences. Desires to be alone. Dislikes company and consolation.

Tendency to morbidity; long-lasting grief; tearful; easily startled. Worse for sympathy and consolation. Misplaced affections. Sensitive to the sun. Very sensitive to noise and music. Drops things from nervous weakness. Great emaciation, losing flesh while eating well. Throat and neck emaciate more rapidly than the rest of the body. Cannot pass urine in the presence of other people or nurse. Craves salt. Dislikes fat and bread, also slimy substances such as oysters. Unquenchable thirst. Tissues appear to hold more fluid than is normal.

Headache. Headache in school-children. Blinding pain as though a thousand hammers were knocking on the brain. Worse on awakening in the morning. After menses. Before attack, numbness and tingling in lips, tongue and nose, relieved by sleep.

Colds and Coughs. Patient catches cold very easily, and repeatedly. Violent fluent coryza for first few days and then watery albuminous discharge and violent sneezing. It is followed by stoppage of nose, with difficulty in breathing and loss of smell and taste. (Very often a homoeopath uses *Nat. mur.* which infallibly stops cold that starts with sneezing. Whether this is a wise procedure is doubtful, as it may cause a suppression of discharge.)

Fever. Chill between 9 and 11 a.m. with violent thirst, which increases with fever and heat. Coldness of the body and marked continued chilliness. Sweats on every exertion. Constipation. Loss of appetite. Fever blisters like pearls about the lips.

Menstruation. Irregular, and very often profuse menstruation. Bearing down pains, headaches and backaches. Better for pressure. Worse in the morning. Hot during menses.

Skin. Oily, greasy, especially on hairy parts. Urticaria after violent exercise, itch and burn. Warts on palm of hands. Worse eating salt and at the seashore.

Worse — 9-11 a.m. Lying down (gets bored). Writing, reading, mental exertion and talking. Salt. From sea air, heat of sun or stove. Closed rooms. (Very often on tube trains he feels sudden desire for fresh air, but once in fresh air he feels chilly and cold.)

Better — In open air. Lying on right side. Cold bathing. Pressure against back. Lying on something hard. Loosening of tight clothing.

Compare: *Sal marinum.*

Complementary: *Apis, Sepia, Thuja.*
Antidotes: *Arsenicum, Phosphorus,* but can be administered before
   these.

NOTE: Do not repeat very often without an intercurrent remedy
called for by the symptoms, in chronic cases. It should never be given
during a fever paroxysm.

Natrum sulphuricum (Sulphate of Sodium — Glauber's Salt)
Indicated remedy for complaints due to living in damp places, also
severe exposure to the sun.

Characteristics: Patient like a barometer. Feels every change of weather
from dry to wet. Forecasts rain or storm. Hates sea air and even
seaweed. Sad and melancholy particularly when the weather is dull
or rainy. Periodic attacks of mania. Depressed. Cries on listening
to music. Suicidal tendency, especially in the morning. Must exercise
restraint not to shoot himself! Inability to think, especially in the
morning. Dislikes talking or being spoken to. Timid, anxious, with
loss of interest in everything. 'All-goneness', empty sensation in the
chest. Must hold chest for support. Dreams of running water. Thirsty
for something cold.

Shock. The remedy for ill-effects of falls and injuries to the head and
chest, especially in slight concussion. Muzziness and all conditions
arising as a result of such injuries.

Chest. Great soreness of chest, more often on the left side, during
cough. Has to sit up in bed and hold his chest with both hands.
Empty feeling in chest. Catarrhs with greenish-yellow mucus — often
after-effects of dampness, e.g. walking in a storm, living in a damp
place, often damp beds and damp basements.

Digestive System. Duodenal catarrh. Sour vomiting of bile. Liver sore
to touch. Sharp stitching pains. Cannot bear tight clothes round
waist. On first rising in the morning, he has sudden and severe urge
to pass a stool which is gushing, loose, yellow and full of flatus.
Involuntary stools when passing wind. All abdominal conditions
caused by over-effects of sun. Rheumatic conditions caused as in chest
conditions, swellings of joints fluctuating with dampness and electrical
atmospheres. Every spring the patient's rheumatism and hay fever
return.
Worse —   Damp weather. In damp houses. From getting wet. At
            the seashore. Bad effects of the sun. More often worse

on left side. Lying on left side. Undressing, especially with his skin symptoms.

Better — Dry weather. Pressure. Changing position.

Compare: *Natrum mur.*, *Sulph.*

Nux vomica (Poison-nut)

An old remedy, but useful for many of the conditions incidental to modern life.

Characteristics: Typical *Nux vomica* patient is rather thin, active, nervous and irritable. Leads indoor and sedentary life. Does a good deal of mental work with mental strain. Needs stimulus of coffee, wine, tobacco, drugs, etc. possibly in excess. There are two types, one the practical, irrational, highly intelligent, zealous, quick tempered, over-eating and drinking type. The other romantic, over-sexed, over-drinking, a tyrant during the day, a debaucher at night. Both types are wonderful 'providers' but difficult to get on with. It is mainly a male remedy. He exaggerates but does not invent his illnesses. Very good sense of smell, all senses are acute. Despises games, faints easily. Cannot bear an offence to his pride or dignity. Cannot bear things out of place. Predominantly a meat-eater. *Nux vomica* is the best remedy for the bad effects of coffee, alcohol, tobacco, highly spiced or seasoned food, and over eating.

Headache. Headache over the eyes. Vertigo. Brain feels turning in a circle. Scalp sensitive. Frontal headache, with desire to press hard against something. Intoxicated feeling, worse in the morning, from mental exertion, alcohol and tobacco, over-eating. Headache in sunshine. Head feels distended and sore after debauch. Best remedy for a hangover.

Colds. Nose stuffed up, especially at night. Coryza, fluent in day time. Stuffy cold after exposure to dry cold atmosphere.

Coughs and Sore Throat. Sensation of roughness, tightness and tension. Tonsils red. Worse swallowing. Uvula swollen, stitches into the ear. Cough caused during inspiration. Worse in warm room or coming into a warm room. Cough in the evening and when asleep. Dry in the evening, loose in the morning. Discharges thick bland yellowish-green. Better from cold fresh air. Wants door thrown open.

Stomach — Digestive Disorders. Pain in stomach after eating. Indigestion. Sour bitter nausea and vomiting. Constant nausea with feeling 'I would be so much better if only I could vomit'. Cannot bear tight clothes. Difficult belching of gas. Feeling of having eaten too much. Food rises into mouth. Rumbling and gurgling in abdomen. Colic. Worse in bed. Pressure as of stone several hours after eating.

Diarrhoea. Diarrhoea after a debauch, worse in the morning. Ptomaine poisoning. Diarrhoea after consumption of tinned food. Movements in intestines before every stool. Watery diarrhoea at night. Discharge of green mucus, evacuations of mucus only. Stools relieve pain for a while.

Menstruation. Too early, profuse and lasts too long. Irregular. Easy fainting before menstruation. Pain in sacrum, with desire for stool and frequent urination.

Influenza. Chilly in warm room. Cold creeps in back. Perspiration sour, only one side of the body. Profuse morning sweat. Feels as if hot water has been thrown over him. Palpitations with anxiety. Dry cough at night relieved on sitting up, returns on lying down. Thirstless, no hunger. Tearful. Peevish. Craves sympathy. Aching in limbs and back, and gastric symptoms. Chilly, must be covered in every stage of fever. Chilliness on being uncovered, yet he does not want to be covered up again.

Useful remedy for the cramps.

Worse — Morning. Mental exertion. After eating. Touch. Spices. Stimulants. Narcotics. Dry weather. Cold.

Better — From a nap, if allowed to finish it. In evening. While at rest. Damp, wet weather. Strong pressure.

Compare: *Kali carb., Bry., Sepia.*

Complementary: *Lyc., Sepia, Sulphur.*

Antidotes: *Zinc.* Many remedies and drugs, especially *Coff., Ignatia, Cocc.*

Phosphorus (Phosphorus)

Characteristics: The burning adolescent; a butterfly who is easily 'enthused' for anything that comes his way. Magnetically sensitive; the 'cheerful clairvoyant' who is refined to a state of degeneracy. He wants to change his ideas but not his hats! He does not want to steady himself. Abstraction of mind, answers questions irrelevantly, or refuses to answer. Understands the question only after repeating it. Difficult concentration. Anxiety when alone, hence a fear of being alone. Loathing of life. Sadness in the evening. Sensitive to light. No staying power or resistance. Suddenly affectionate. Generally symptoms from sexual excesses. Burning in the palms of hands often precipitated by emotional upsets, such as grief. Headaches are relieved by eating, while the patient in himself is getting worse. Extreme hunger a day or two before an acute illness. During pregnancy is unable to drink water, sight of it causes vomiting. Desires large quantities of cold drinks which make him sick as soon as they get warm in the stomach. Craves salt, likes cold meals, must eat often or he faints.

Headache. Heat coming from the spine reaches the head and the patient gets headaches which are improved by eating, and application of cold water.

Eyes. Sees better in twilight. Unable to bear light. Congestion. Enlarged blood vessels. Sees a green halo round a candle-light. Letters appear red. Eyes red, burn, smart, worse for cold applications.

Ears. Hearing difficult, especially the human voice. Sounds re-echo.

Nose. Chronic catarrh, with small haemorrhages.

Throat and Chest. Painful hoarseness, which is worse on speaking, and in the evening. Larynx very painful, cannot talk on account of pain. Cough worse in cold air, reading, laughing and talking. Cough hard, tight, racking. Tightness across the chest with great weight on chest. Whole body trembles with cough. Sputum rusty, blood red or purulent. Nervous cough provoked by strong odours, worse in presence of strangers and in a cold room.

Fever. Chilly every evening. Cold knees at night. A dynamic with lack of thirst, but unnatural hunger. Hectic, with small quick pulse. Viscid, sticky night sweats. Stupid delirium. Profuse perspiration.

Worse — Weather changes. In cold. In thunderstorms (knows when they are coming). Inhalation of cold air. In the morning. Eating. Eating warm food. Salt. Emissions. Exertion. Being alone in the dark.

Better — Being rubbed or mesmerized. Warmth generally.

Complementary: *Ars., Cepa., Lyc., Silica.*

Phos. antidotes nausea and vomiting from chloroform and ether.

Pulsatilla (Wind Flower)

A plant that grows in sandy soil and blooms at Easter. A wind flower, supposed to have been cultivated from the tears of Venus. A weather-cock remedy.

Characteristics: A mild, lachrymose, slow, phlegmatic temperament. Good-tempered, mild and yielding, especially when in normal health. Frivolous and good-humouredly vague. Sometimes stubborn, but passively so. A tendency towards grief, and silent peevishness. Jealous, touchy, emotionally sensitive. Weepy, hysterical, easily moved by external influences. Religious mania. Fanatical, in their queer, particular, innocent way. Self-pitying 'Nobody understands me or does what I do'. Greatly dependent and dependable. Yield very quickly and do what they are told. Easily persuaded into sex, often against their own will. Never pugnacious. Sympathetic and crave for sympathy. Fear of dark, of ghosts, of being alone, and death. Fear of opposite sex. Homosexual. When there is a real sorrowful mental shock they stand it well. Like to be out of doors. Desire for fresh air. Chilly, but averse to heat. Mouth is dry but there is no thirst. One-sided complaints. One hand cold, the other warm. They sweat on one side only. Cannot sleep in the evening or first part of night, but sleep late in the morning. Weaker the longer they sleep. It is not predominantly a woman's remedy, but is often used in female cases, because it has a marked effect on the female genital tract. Invaluable in confinements. Uterine inertia. It is the picture of plump fair people, who gradually become darker. Physically inert through lack of vitality. Apt to be lazy. Abuse of tea or coffee. Inclined to eat things that do not agree with her. Averse to butter and fat. Rheumatic pains wander from joint to joint. Better with gentle movement. Drawing erratic pains. Symptoms change. Feels cold, yet better for cool air. Female discharges, bland, thick yellow or greenish, non-irritating.

Sleeplessness. Wide-awake in the evening, does not want to go to bed. Restless. Sleep before midnight is prevented by fixed idea, or recurrent melody, or too many thoughts crowding into mind. Unable to sleep after late supper. Weeping because she could not sleep. Characteristic position for sleeping with arms overhead. Sound asleep when it is time to get up.

Headache. Throbbing congested hot head. Better for cold applications, and walking slowly in the open air. Headaches connected with menstruation or suppressed menstruation. Periodic sick headache, vomits sour food. Headaches from over-eating, from ice cream. Thirstless. Weeps easily. Changeable. Must have fresh air. Worse for heat.

Eyes. Excellent remedy for styes with thick, creamy, virulent discharge. Conjunctivitis. Sand in the eye. Itching in the eye and around the eye.

Toothache. Itching of teeth. Worse on taking anything warm in the mouth, better on cold applications or drinking cold water, better in open air, worse from warmth. Toothache of children with summer diarrhoea and bowel disorders.

Colds. One of our sheet-anchors in conditions of catarrh with loss of smell. Thick yellow discharge. Better in the open air. Stuffing up of the nose at night, and in the house, copious flow in the morning and in the open air.

Stomach. Gastric troubles from over-eating, rich food, ice cream, etc. Tongue heavily coated. Mouth may be full of mucus and yet it feels dry. Lips swollen. Constipation alternating with diarrhoea. Symptoms constantly change, even no two stools are alike.

Menstruation. Particularly suitable when menstruation is late. A high dose will set a missing period correct. As it does not induce abortion, it may be used as a test for absent periods where pregnancy is suspected.

Sunstroke. A useful remedy for ailments caused from the heat of the sun. Excessive vertigo. Headache with throbbing in the brain.

Apoplexy. Unconscious. Face purplish and bloated. Violent beating of heart. Pulse collapse.

Influenza. Coldness. Chilliness begins in back. Temperature rises rapidly. Great heat with profuse sweat, but sweat does not cause fall in temperature. Useful remedy to help with post-influenzal depression or weakness.

Worse —   From twilight to midnight. Before storms. Lying on left side. Lying on painless side. With feet hanging down. Warm room. Warm coverings. Fatty food. Abuse of tea.

Better —   In open air. Motion. Cold applications. Cold food. Cold drinks. After eating. After a good cry.

Compare: *Silica, Sulphur, Kali bich., Kali sulph.*

Complementary: *Coffea, Nux vom.*

Pyrogenium (Artificial Sepsin)
Characteristics: Pyrogenium is the great remedy for septic states with intense restlessness. All discharges are horribly offensive. Great pain

and violent burning in abscesses. Patient loquacious. Thinks he is wealthy. Feels as if crowded with arms and legs. Cannot tell whether he is dreaming while awake or asleep. Restless. Aches all over, relieved by tossing about. Life-saving remedy in severe infectious diseases when the best selected remedy fails to improve.

Colds. Severe suppurating quinsies with dirty, offensive smell from the mouth.

Influenza (Breakbone fever). Coldness and chilliness. Chill begins in the back. Temperature rises rapidly. Great heat with profuse hot sweat, but sweating does not cause a fall in temperature. Aching in all limbs and bones. Bed feels too hard. Constipation with complete inertia. Patient sleeps deep and comatose in a dream state all night. Better from motion.
Complementary: *Bryonia.*
Do not repeat remedy very frequently.
Master remedy for severe, acute, sudden food (especially bad meat) poisoning, with vomiting the colour of coffee grounds. Severe pain in the left chest and griping pains in the stomach with collapse, sweating and an acute septic state. It is also a master remedy for septic states in puerperium (Mothers who have delivered a baby recently) when the symptoms are of an acute severe septicaemia.

Rhus toxicodendron (Poison Ivy)
Frequently indicated for its effects on the skin, rheumatic pains, cartilage and articular surface pains, mucous membrane affections and a typhoid-type of fever. *Rhus* affects fibrous tissues markedly, joints, tendons and sheaths.

Characteristics: Painful swelling of joints — pains which are worse for rest, better for movement. Tearing pain, mainly associated with rheumatism. Ailments from strains, sprains, over-lifting, getting wet while perspiring. Tearing asunder pains, especially in cold weather. Mental restlessness, anxiety, apprehension. Great apprehension at night. Dreams of great exertion, rowing, swimming, working hard at his daily occupation. Fears he will die of being poisoned. Cannot remain in bed. Must constantly change his position to obtain physical relief. Thoughts of suicide. Sadness. Listlessness. Brain feels loose, as if struck against skull on rising and walking. Unquenchable thirst, desire for milk. No appetite for any kind of food.

Sleeplessness. Due to pain of rheumatic type leading to sleepless nights.

Due to bruises, etc. also injury to the eyes. Restless at night, has to change position frequently. Cannot remain in bed. Dreams of labour, running, marching, rushing.

Headache. Feels as if a board were strapped on the forehead. Heavy head. Stupefied as if intoxicated. Brain feels loose, and seems to fall against side of skull. Brain loaded. Scalp sensitive. Vertigo when rising.

Eyes. Injuries to the eye. Intensive ulceration to the cornea.

Ears. Pains in the ear. Feeling as if there is something in them. Discharge of bloody pus.

Mouth. Jaws crack when chewing. Teeth feel long and loose. Tongue coated except for red triangle at tip. Bitter taste.

Colds. Violent coryza. Mouth, throat and nose blocked up every evening. Thirst for cold drinks, especially at night. Cold drinks bring on chilliness and cough. Worse for being uncovered. Bones ache. Sneezing and coughing, worse in the evening and at night. Tickling behind upper part of sternum.

Chest and Coughs. Dry, teasing cough. Worse from midnight to morning, from being uncovered, or even putting a hand out of bed. Cough during sleep. Hoarseness from over-straining voice. Patient feels better for talking or singing. Worse in cold wet weather. Restless. Must move.

Stomach. Drowsiness after eating. Violent abdominal pain. Better lying on the abdomen. Bitter taste in mouth.

Stools. Frothy painless stools. Cadaverous odour. Suppuration process near the rectum, like infected piles.

Influenza. Stiff and bruised on first morning. This passes off with movement, but he becomes weak and must rest. Suffering worse when still, and kept without motion. Worse in cold damp weather, and if left cold and damp after perspiring. Anxiety, fear, restlessness, worse at night. Weeps without knowing why. Fear of poison. Severely aching bones. Thirst. Perspiration.

Menstruation. Menses early, profuse, prolonged and acrid. Pains shooting upwards in vagina. Better from movement. Worse from hot bath, hot water bottle, while washing parts.

Skin. Surface raw. Oozes with an offensive smell. Much burning and itching. Eruptions, thick crusts, made worse by rubbing.

Worse — Wet rainy weather. Before a storm. Change of weather. At night, especially after midnight. During cold. During rest. Getting wet after perspiration. When lying on back or on right side. Worse at 5 a.m. and 5 p.m.

Better — Warm dry weather. Movement. Walking. Change of position. Stretching out limbs. Rubbing. Heat. Food.

NOTE: When *Rhus tox.* is administered as an acute remedy, do not let the patient have very hot baths, as it stops the action.

Complementary: *Bryonia, Calc. fluor., Phytolacca.*
Inimical: *Apis.*

Ruta graveolens (Rue-bitterwort)
Acts upon the periosteum and cartilages, eyes and uterus. Lameness after sprains. Complaints of sprain of flexor tendons. Overstrain of eye muscles. All parts of the body are painful, as if bruised. Legs give out on rising from a chair, hips and thighs feel weak. Feeling of intense lassitude, weakness and despair. Injured 'bruised' bones. Pain and stiffness in wrists and hands. Thighs ache when stretching the limbs. Pain in bones of feet and ankles. Contraction of fingers. Sciatica.

Headache and Eyes. Eye strain followed by headache. Eyes red and painful from sewing or reading. Disturbance of accommodation. Headache from too many intoxicating drinks. Pain in night-reading examinee eyes. Also night worker's headaches and eye strain.

Cough. Cough with copious thick yellow expectoration. Chest feels weak. Painful spot on sternum. Short of breath with tightness of chest.

Stools. Constipation, alternating with frothy mucous stools. Discharge of blood with stool. Tearing stitches in rectum when sitting. A large stool evacuated with difficulty as from loss of peristaltic action of rectum. Frequent urging to stool but only rectum prolapses. Slightest stooping or crouching down causes rectum to protrude.

Worse — Lying down. From cold. From wet weather.
Compare: *Arnica, Rhus, Silica, Phyt., Jaborandi.*
Complementary: *Calc. phos.*
Antidote: *Camphor.*

Silica (Pure Flint — a hard stone)
Silica is found in the stalks of grain or grass, and gives them the

resistance and capacity to stand upright.

Characteristics: A chilly, tidy, neat, orderly person, with a neat little body. Very often gifted, but shy and timid, with no resistance or protection within. Exhaustion and 'brain-fag' in professional people and businessmen. Mental labour very difficult. Anxious. Yielding. Sensitive to all impressions. Hates noise, is easily startled. Cries when spoken to. Dislikes taking risks. Has fixed ideas. Tries to study and steady himself, but cannot do so. Excessive thirst. Dislikes meat and warm food. Wants plenty of warm clothes. Sits close to fire. Hates draughts. Often suffers from deficiencies of nutrition, not from lack of food, but because of failure to assimilate. Tendency to form scars where there should be none. Cuts suppurate. Ripens abscesses, since it promotes suppurations, especially long-lasting, of glands and joints. Low potencies mature abscesses and heal after discharge. The phase between *Hepar sulph.* and *Silica* should be very carefully considered.

Headache. Pain from mental exertion. Dizziness and vertigo when looking up. Offensive sweating of the head extends to the neck. Better from warm applications and wrapping up the head. Worse in cold damp weather. Worse in change of weather.

Coughs and Colds. Colds occur one after another. Thin, watery, yellowish, offensive discharge. Pricking feeling, as if pin in tonsil. Parotid glands swollen. Cough and sore throat, spitting out little granules with an offensive odour, bloody or purulent. Worse lying down; suppurative stages of cough.

Skin. Offensive sweating and suppuration between toes. Useful in Athlete's Foot. Icy cold feet. Whitlows, abscesses, boils. Broken nails.

Worse — At the new moon. In cold wind. Damp. Cold. Uncovering. Lying down. Lying on left side. During menstruation. From washing.

Better — In summer. From warmth. In wet humid weather. Wrapping up of head.

Compare: *Hepar, Picric Acid, Kali phos., Hypericum, Ruta, Sanic.*
Complementary: *Thuja, Sanic., Puls., Fluor Acid* which may be indicated when a *Silica* patient does not respond any more to *Silica*. A single dose restarts the action of *Silica*.
Mercurius and *Silica* do not follow each other.

Spongia tosta (Roasted Sponge)
Characteristics: Men, women and children with tubercular diathesis.

Light-haired, lean, thin, weak, withered persons. Anxiety, fear, worse after sleep, fear of death; of the future; that something might happen. Marked anxiety and terror in nearly all complaints. Palpitation, with anxiety and suffocation after midnight, before and during menses.

Headache. Rush of blood to the neck and head. Paroxysms of the head, with anxiety and suffocation.

Throat. Thyroid glands swollen, with choking attacks at night.

Coughs. Dry, raw, sibilant cough, with no mucus. Worse for sweets, cold drinks, smoking, reading aloud, singing, talking, swallowing, cold dry winds. Attacks of croup during inspiration, worse before midnight.
Worse — Before noon. Before midnight. Lying down. Ascending.
Compare: *Aconite, Lachesis., Merc. prot. iod.*

Staphysagria (Stavesacre)
Characteristics: Very sensitive type of person. Impetuous. Melancholic. Sad. Prefers solitude. Petulant. Sensitive to what is said about him. Dwells on old insults and things done in the past. Dwells on sexual matters. Remedy for nervous afflictions with irritability. Ill-effects from anger and sexual sins and excesses. Patient worse after grief and anger. Worse by least touch on affected parts. Loss of fluids. Better after breakfast or rest at night. Remedy for nervousness after extraction of teeth. Diseases of the urinary tract. Sleeps all day long. Body aches all over and cannot sleep. Cannot sleep for sexual anxiety. Styes and backaches keep the patient awake.

Headache. Stupefying headaches. Better from yawning. Brain feels squeezed. Sensation as if head full of lead. Very often accompanied by itching above and behind the ears. Headaches of sexual frustration.

Eyes. Excellent remedy for styes in the eye. Lacerated wounds of the cornea. Itching of eyelids. Bursting pain in the eyeballs.

Stomach. Canine hunger even when stomach is full. Nausea after abdominal operation. Craving for tobacco.

Urinary Tract. Important remedy for cystitis of the newly married. Repeated urination. Burning in the urethra. Urging and pain after urination especially in some newly-married women — they get a severe ineffectual urge to urinate. This is partly out of nervousness and clumsy consummation; from nervousness over the new relationship as a whole, and from bruising of virginal parts. Worse after grief or anger. Better after rest at night.

Useful remedy when injuries are caused by sharp instruments, glass, etc. and also for neuralgia after surgical operations. (Also *Hypericum*.)

Also useful for toothache during menstruation. Toothache worse from the touch of food or liquid, and biting and chewing.

Worse — Anger. Indignation. Grief. Mortification. Loss of fluids. Sexual excess. Tobacco. Least touch on affected parts.

Better — After breakfast. Warmth. Rest at night.

Compare: *Ignatia*.

Complementary: *Caust., Ferrum., Pyro.*

Antidotes: *Camph., Coffea.*

Urtica urens (Stinging-nettle)

Is one of the finest remedies for burns and scalds. Also useful in certain skin diseases. Itching blotches. Urticaria, burning heat with blistering. Violent itching. Nettle-rash. Patient is worse from touch, cold moist air, and water.

Is also a useful remedy for the ill-effects of eating shellfish. Rheumatism associated with urticaria-like eruptions. Neuritis associated with such conditions.

Tinctures and lotions are extremely useful in burns.

Shock. Useful remedy for shock from burns or scalds.

Worse — Cold moist air. Water. Snow. Touch.

Compare: *Medusa, Nat. mur., Lac. can., Rhus, Apis, Puls., Lycop., Bombyx, Chloral, Astac.*

BIBLIOGRAPHY

General
Aurobindo, Sri, *The Synthesis of Yoga*: Aurobindo Ashram, Pondicherry.
Bhattacharyya, Dr B., *The Science of Tridosha*: Gotham Book, New York.
Bennett, J. G., *The Dramatic Universe*. (4 vols): Hodder, London.
Bennett, J. G., *Energies*.
Bennett, J. G., *Transformation*. Coombe Springs Press.
Elliott, R., *Not Just a Load of Old Lentils*: White Eagle Pub., Liss, Hants.
Jaffrey, Madhur, *Eastern Vegetarian Cooking*: Cape, London. Published in the USA by Knopf, N.Y. as *World of the East Vegetarian Cooking*.
Jung, C. G., *Modern Man in Search of a Soul*: Routledge, London/Harcourt Brace Janovich Inc., San Diego.
Jung, C. G., *Four Archetypes*: Routledge, London/Harcourt Brace Janovich Inc., San Diego.
Jung, C. G., *Synchronicity*: Routledge, London/Princeton University Press.
Ornstein, Robert E., *The Psychology of Consciousness*: W. H. Freeman, London/Penguin Books N.Y.

Homoeopathy for the Beginner
British Homoeopathic Association, *Guide to Homoeopathy*: London.
Shepherd, *Treatment of Cats*: Health Science Press.
Shepherd, *Treatment of Dogs*: Health Science Press.
Woods, F., *Homoeopathy in the Nursery*: Brit. Hom. Ass., London.

Intermediate
Borland, Dr Douglas, *Children's Types*: Brit. Hom. Ass., London.
Gibson, *Elements of Homoeopathy*: Brit. Hom. Ass., London.
Hobhouse, R., *Christian Samuel Hahnemann*: Daniel.
Puddephat, *How to Find the Correct Remedy*: Health Science Press.
Woods, F., *Essentials of Homoeopathic Prescribing with Rapid Recovery*: Health Science Press.

Textbooks for the Advanced Student
Allen, *Keynotes of Leading Remedies*: Boericke, Philadelphia.
Bidwell, *How to use the Repertory*: Health Science Press.
Clarke, *Dictionary of Materia Medica*: Health Science Press.
Gibson, *First Aid Homoeopathy*: Brit. Hom. Ass., London.
Hahnemann, S., *Organon of Medicine*: Jain Pubs., New Delhi.
Jain Pubs., *Regional Leaders in Hom. Therapeutics*: New Delhi.
Kent, Dr J. T., *Lectures on Homoeopathic Philosophy*: Thorsons, Wellingborough.
Shepherd, *Homoeopathy in Epidemic Diseases*: Health Science Press.
Shepherd, *Homoeopathy for the First Aider*: Health Science Press.
Tyler, M. L., *Homoeopathic Drug Pictures*: Health Science Press.
Tyler, M. L. and Weir, J., *Repertorising*: Brit. Hom. Ass., London.
Wadia, D S. R., *What is Homoeopathy?*: Horn Publishers, Bombay.
Weir, J., *Homoeopathy a System of Therapeutics*: Brit. Hom. Ass., London.
Weir, J., *Hahnemann on Homoeopathic Philosophy*: Brit. Hom. Ass., London.
Weir, J., *Cases Illustrating the Homoeopathic Philosophy*: Brit. Hom. Ass., London.
Wheeler, C., *An Introduction to the Principles and Practice of Homoeopathy*: Health Science Press.

For the Qualified Practitioner
Nash, Dr E. B., *Regional Leaders in Homoeopathic Therapeutics*: Health Science Press.

Tyler, M. L. and Weir J., *Acute Conditions, Injuries, etc*: Brit. Hom. Ass., London.
The Pointers (Keynote symptoms for medicines for use in specific conditions): Brit. Hom. Ass., London.

No 1 Colds, acute chests.
    2 Stomach, digestive disorders.
    3 Dentition, rickets.
    4 Convulsion, rheumaticism, chorea.
    5 Zymotic Diseases, typhoid.
    6 Drugs of strong mentality.
    7 Nephritis, suppression.
    8 Vertigo, sunstroke, headache.
    9 Some organ remedies.

Allen, Dr J. H., *Chronic Miasms*: A. Ray, Bombay.
Bell, J. B., *The Homoeopathic Therapeutics of Diarrhoea*: Boericke, Philadelphia.
Boenninghausen's Therapeutic Pocket Book: Boericke, Philadelphia.
Boericke, Dr Wm., *Materia Medica and Repertory*: Boericke, Philadelphia.
Boger, Dr C. M., *Synoptic Key of the Materia Medica*: B. Jain Pubs, New Delhi.
Borland, Dr Douglas, *Influenza*: Brit. Hom. Ass., London.
Coulter, *Homoeopathic Medicine*: American Foundation for Homoeopathy.
Farrington, *Clinical Materia Medica*: A. Roy and Co., Bombay.
Gladstone Clarke, G., *De Cachords*: A. Nelson and Co., London.
Homoeopathic Publishing Company, *Clinical Repertory to Clarke's Dictionary of Materia Medica*: London.
Hahnemann, S., *Chronic Diseases — Their Peculiar Nature and their Homoeopathic Cure* (2 vols): B. Jain Publications, New Delhi.
Kent, Dr J. T., *Repertory*: B. Jain Pubs., New Delhi.
Phatek, *Concise Repertory of Homoeopathic Remedies*: A. Roy and Co., Bombay.
Roberts, H. A., *The Principles and Art of Cure by Homoeopathy*: Health Science Press.
Wadia, Dr S. R., *Horn in Skin Disease*: Horn Medical Pubs., Bombay.

Natural Medicine
Clement, M., *Aluminium, Menace to Health*: Clark and Son, London.
Cunning, A. B. and Innes, F. R., *We are What We Eat*: Salvationist Pub., London.
Biochemical Individuality: The Basis for the Genetotrophic Concept: N/Y Wiley.
General Nutrition Corporation: 418 Ward St., Pittsburg.
Luke, Dr T. D., *Manual of Nature Therapy*: John Wright and Sons Ltd., London.
McCarrison, Sir Robert and Sinclair, H. M., *Nutrition and Health*: Faber, London.
Nutricol: Vitamin Quota, 880 Broadway, New York.
Roddie, J., *Physiology for Practitioners*: Churchill Livingstone, Edinburgh.
Rusholm, P., *Country Medicines*: Health Science Press.
Sams, C., *About Macrobiotics*: Thorsons, Wellingborough.
Stein, Mendel, *Vitamins*: Churchill Livingstone, Edinburgh.
Turner, *Naturopathic First Aid*: Health Science Press.
Williams, R. J., *Nutrition against Diseases*: Pitman, New York.
Williams, R. J., *Nutrition and Alcoholism*: Pitman, New York.
Yudkin, J., *Patterns and Trends in Carbohydrate and their Relation to Disease*: Progressive Nutrition Soc., New York.

USEFUL ADDRESSES

Australia
The Australian Natural Therapies Association (ANTA) is a National body which has been formed to train and unite Naturopaths, regulate standards, and control the industry. The ANTA describe a Natural Therapist as a person who practices one or more of the following: Mineral/Vitamin Therapy, Herbalism, Homoeopathy, Chiropractice, Osteopathy and Acupuncture. Branches are as follows:

ANTA
PO Box 522, Sutherland, N.S.W. 2232

ANTA
Good Health Clinic, 42 Thomas Drive, Chevron Island, Qld. 4217

ANTA
29 Charles Street, South Perth, W.A. 6151

ANTA
289 Cross Road, Clarence Gardens, S.A. 5039

ANTA
49 White Avenue, East Kew, Vic. 3102

ANTA
PO Box 117, Cremorne, N.S.W. 2090

JANTOR (Journal of the Australian Natural Therapies Association)
1st Floor, Block Arcade, 284 Collins Street, Melbourne, Vic. 3000

New Zealand
NZ DIATETIC ASSOC. & NUTRITION SOCY.
PO Box 2607, Christchurch

NZ HOMOEOPATHIC SOCIETY INC.
Box 2939, Auckland

USA
THE UNITED STATES HOMEOPATHIC ASSOCIATION
6560 Backlick Road, Suite 211, Springfield, VA 22150

THE FOUNDATION FOR HOMEOPATHIC EDUCATION & RESEARCH
5916 Chabot Crest, Oakland, CA 94618

HOMEOPATHIC EDUCATIONAL SERVICES
2124 Kittredge Street, Berkeley, CA 94704

NATIONAL CENTER FOR HOMEOPATHY
1500 Massachusetts Avenue, NW, Washington DC 20005

INTERNATIONAL FOUNDATION FOR HOMEOPATHY
1141 NW Market, Seattle, WA 98107

AMERICAN ASSOCIATION FOR HOMEOPATHIC PHARMACISTS
P.O. Box 2273, Falls Church, VA 22072

Canada

THE HOMEOPATHIC SOCIETY OF ALBERTA
P.O. Box 8032, Stn 'F', Edmonton, Alberta, Canada T6H 4N9

CANADIAN NATUROPATHIC ASSOCIATION
259 Midpark Way, Suite 306, Calgary, Alberta, Canada T2X 1M2

ONTARIO COLLEGE OF NATUROPATHIC MEDICINE
43 Benton Street, Kitchener, Ontario, Canada N2G 3H1

INSTITUT NATUROPATHIQUE
1537 Rue Balleray, Longueuil, Quebec, Canada J4M 1S3

HOMEOPATHIC TRAINING PROGRAM
Department of Continuing Education, University of Quebec at Hull,
118 Notre Dame Street, Hull, Quebec, Canada J8X 3S9

PHYSICIANS HOMEOPATHIC SOCIETY OF BRITISH COLUMBIA
20787 Fraser Highway, Langley, British Columbia, Canada V3A 4G4

HOMEOPATHY AND RESEARCH INSTITUTE OF CANADA INC.
Suite 202, 2835 Chemin Gomin Saint Foi, Quebec, Canada G1V 2K1

CANADIAN ACADEMY OF HOMEOPATHIC MEDICINES
10762 82nd Avenue, Edmonton, Alberta, Canada T6E 2A8

UK

THE ACADEMY OF CLASSICAL HOMOEOPATHY
16 St Michael's Mount, Northampton

THE SOCIETY OF HOMOEOPATHS
101 Sebastian Avenue, Shenfield, Brentwood, Essex CM15 8PP

THE HOMOEOPATHIC DEVELOPMENT FOUNDATION
Harcourt House, 19a Cavendish Square, London W1M 9AD

THE BRITISH HOMOEOPATHIC ASSOCIATION
27a Devonshire Street, London W1N 1RJ

THE HAHNEMANN SOCIETY
Humane Education Centre, Avenue Lodge, Bounds Green Road, London N22 4EU

THE BRITISH HOLISTIC MEDICAL ASSOCIATION
179 Gloucester Place, London NW1 6DX

CCAM (Council for Complementary and Alternative Medicine)
10 Belgrave Square, London SW1X 8PH

THE FACULTY OF HOMOEOPATHY
Hahnemann House, Powis Place, Great Ormond Street, London WC1N 3HT

General Index

Index of Homoeopathic Remedies